Unworthy Weight

Reclaiming Your Worth from a Number on a Scale and Finding True Identity in Christ

Kristin Williams
RDN, LD, CEDRD

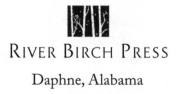

RIVER BIRCH PRESS

Daphne, Alabama

Scripture quotations are taken from *THE HOLY BIBLE: New International Version* ©1978 by the New York International Bible Society, used by permission of Zondervan Bible Publishers.

ISBN 978-1-951561-21-5
For Worldwide Distribution
Printed in the U.S.A.

River Birch Press
P.O. Box 868
Daphne, Alabama 36526

Table of Contents

To Carol Park:
You are the reason I decided to become a dietitian.

To my husband, parents and sister:
Thank you for believing in me, supporting me
and cheering me on along the way.

To anyone who ever has or ever will struggle
with disordered eating:
This one is for you.

Acknowledgments

Writing this book has been on my heart for many years. I am so grateful for the journey and for the opportunity to share this message with all of my readers. God has ignited a passion within me in the area of body image and helping others to see themselves the way Christ sees them. This is a daily reminder to me, and I am thankful for the platform to share this convicting reminder with others. I pray that the glory is to God and that I make much of Him rather than much of me.

When I was diagnosed with anorexia nervosa at age 13 years old, I had no idea what a dietitian was. Thank you, Carol Park, for being a part of my treatment team and my recovery journey. I will never forget the impact you had on me, and I am forever grateful that God has used you to direct my own career path all these years later. Your work matters.

Jay, thank you for believing in me and supporting me in my passions to pursue private practice, writing, and public speaking. I could not have done this without your support, and I've felt you backing me up along the way. There were many risks involved with this, and I so appreciate your willingness to take each of those risks we faced. Thank you for believing in me and in this message and for sharing the desire to raise our children with this message instilled in their hearts.

Mom, Dad, and Jessica, thank you for being my #1 fans. From reading every unedited chapter, attending speaking events, encouraging me when I felt discouraged, cheering me on in all of my goals, and babysitting during my sessions with clients, I appreciate it more than you know.

Jessica Setnick, thank you for introducing me to the eating disorder professional world and for giving me a space to belong. Thank you for allowing me to catch a glimpse into the life of a successful eating disorder professional, for mentoring me along the way, and for believing in new dietitians. Your work in the field has been so impactful.

Northwest Bible Church and Grace Community Church, thank you for believing in this message enough to allow conversations in the area of worth, identity, and body image to be started through various ministries in the church. This is a huge issue that the church isn't talking about, and I so appreciate you seeing the importance in starting these much needed conversations amongst believers.

Juleeta Harvey, thank you for being you, for your sweet heart and passion for women's ministries, and for your desire to help break the chains of disordered eating and bondage to poor body image. It has been an honor to serve alongside you.

Laura Gilbert, thank you for being my mentor and a strong example of a godly woman, wife, and mother. Thank you for sharing your writing talent with me and for believing in my own writing talents.

To anyone who ever has or ever will struggle with disordered eating, you are not alone. May you wrestle well and may you find your worth and identity in Christ alone. I am cheering you on.

Introduction

Have you ever believed the lie that you can find your identity in a number on the scale? Or have you thought your waist size determines your worth? Have you chased after numerous fad diets, only to become more depressed, more preoccupied with food, and more disconnected from God? What might it look like to reclaim your worth from a number on a scale by finding your true identity in Christ?

Unworthy Weight: Reclaiming Your Worth from a Number on the Scale and Finding True Identity in Christ discusses the issues of body image and disordered eating. This problem is prevalent among Christians, yet few churches talk about it.

Scripture calls us as believers to be holy, set apart for the glory of God. Yet in the diet culture, we blend right in with the rest of the world.

This book is a journey to discovery of God's Word and what it says about creation, our bodies, and food. Scriptural truth will form the foundation of our nutritional beliefs. We will learn what it means to be a temple of the Holy Spirit, and we will challenge the lies of diet culture.

So take a deep breath. Stop dieting. Stop searching for a number to define your worth.

May you find worth only in Him. Everything else is unworthy weight.

~ One ~

THIS IS MY STORY, THIS IS MY SONG

For twenty-three years, I was at war with my body. I do not remember one day during my adolescent years when I felt comfortable in my own skin.

During summers at the pool, when other third graders were having fun doing cannonballs and playing Marco Polo, I wallowed in shame over my body and wore swim shorts to cover my thighs. I now know that, unfortunately, this is an all-too-familiar struggle for young children. I've watched my niece fight a similar battle as she hides her stomach in a one-piece.

In the grade-school cafeteria, I was embarrassed to eat in front of my peers. I worried what kids might think about my packed lunch and feared they believed I shouldn't eat because I was already too fat.

In middle school, I was a cheerleader and compared my body to others on the squad. I always worried that I stuck out and was too big. I thought I didn't fit in, and I believed my opinion of my body was correct. I coveted the flyer position on the squad. I thought that, if I were skinny, people would want me in that role.

In athletics, I also compared myself to others and never believed I measured up. I felt awkward and round and thought boys would like me if only I looked different.

In eighth grade, I asked a coach to help me get healthy and lose weight. He was a large, muscular man. Imagine Gaston from *Beauty and the Beast* and you have a visual of Coach Suddarth, four dozen raw eggs and all. He gave me some tips and tricks in the name of "health" and never meant harm.

However, this led to an obsession with restrictive behaviors. Combined with many other variables, including a genetic predisposition, my obsession set me up for an eating disorder.

One day, my eighth-grade math teacher pulled my coach to the side and asked what he was doing to me. She knew something wasn't right. Soon the school counselor called me to her office. She asked if I would eat a donut if she offered it. I thought that was a weird question and told her no.

She contacted my parents, addressed her concerns, and asked questions. Eating disorders are tricky. They can easily be disguised as "eating healthier" and "exercising more." My parents were shocked. Living with someone day in and day out, we often don't notice such drastic physical changes.

Before I knew it, I was meeting with a therapist, a registered dietitian, and a pediatric cardiologist, who told me I wasn't eating enough to nourish my big toe. They immediately put me on a meal plan and restricted my exercise, which meant I missed out on a family skiing trip to Canada.

I was forced to swap my cheerleading outfit for a choir-assistant badge. I was only to observe choir rehearsal and not move. In other words, the music teacher babysat me because they didn't know where else to place me during this period.

After a year of weight restoration and therapy, I was "in recovery." I'm thankful the doctor diagnosed my anorexia early, and intervention happened almost immediately. Both decrease the likelihood of relapse.

However, my battle did not end there. In many ways, it had just begun. For years after my diagnosis, I struggled with rebound eating. I felt out of control, overly stuffed, and very much ashamed.

I remember staying the night with friends in the summer

and watching them move on after a couple slices of pizza. Not me. I continued and continued and continued to eat, ravaging the fridge and pantry and making jokes about it along the way, in hopes of hiding or making light of my deep fear of not being able to stop.

No one had told me that restrictive eating could lead to a season of overeating, and so for years, I thought something was wrong with me. Later, I learned that dietary restriction was like pulling back a rubber band. Eventually that band would fly across the room, resulting in out-of-control behaviors.

I remember not having the patience to let a microwave meal heat properly, and so I ate frostbitten lasagna. It seemed easy for my friends to move on with their lives after a meal, but food constantly tormented me. My mind was stuck on what I had just eaten. I wondered whether I'd be able to get more and what I'd need to do the following day to make up for it. This mindset kept me in a diet cycle for years.

I remember seeing how much I could eat after school before my parents got home. One snack led to another, which led to another, all triggered by underlying emotions rather than physical hunger.

I remember babysitting for the preacher's kid and feeling as if I could not stop eating. I sorted through their pantry and tried to arrange boxes and packages to look as though I hadn't eaten as much as I had. I played around with the remaining pizza slices in the box and tried to make it appear as if more remained. But how much pizza could an infant eat? I couldn't blame it on her.

In college, I wanted to work with eating disorders, so I prepared for a career in either dietetics or psychology. Interested in nutrition, I decided to pursue a degree in nutritional sciences and become a dietitian.

My toxic relationship with food followed me to the campus. I was on my own, with groceries to choose and meals to prepare. But I was surrounded by other students who wanted to go out to eat more than I was used to. I planned boring, healthy meals and purchased the entire produce section at the grocery store. But I ended up at Cheddar's on Thursday nights, shoving my face with chips and spinach artichoke dip while my lettuce slowly wilted in the fridge and my bananas browned on the countertop.

I always thought, *Tomorrow will be different. Tomorrow I'll start anew.* And then, due to the stress of school or because I needed the energy to pull an all-nighter, I ate as if tomorrow would never come. Or simply because I viewed certain foods as off limits.

In class, I was surrounded by other dietetic students who took notes while munching on carrot sticks and sugar snap peas. My peers loved to cook for fun and bake gluten-free muffins.

I felt like a fraud as if I didn't fit in. Often I packed a lunch and then met friends at Chick-fil-A instead. How could I ever help people if I couldn't help myself?

During my first year after college, I worked as a diet tech at a local hospital. The diets continued, as did my self-loathing. I asked patients about their appetite while mine was out of control.

The following summer, I was accepted to a dietetic internship at Medical City Dallas Hospital as part of their charter class. I don't know why, but eventually, something started to click. I still struggled with comparison and feeling like a wannabe who didn't have it together. But slowly, something began to change.

Eventually, I became much more mindful and aware of my eating. Little by little, I started learning what it meant to nourish my body and take the morality out of eating. My thoughts changed too. I wasn't as hyper-focused on food and what I had eaten. My body settled to an appropriate size over time, and I began to appreciate my body as never before. This was not by any means an overnight process, but rather a slow season of learning. I've tried to determine the cause, but I can't say one specific event sparked this change within me. All I know is that change is possible, and toxic relationships with food can be healed.

This was a freeing time in my life, but every once in a while, my past still haunted me. I later worked as an outpatient dietitian, providing general nutrition counseling. But at times, I reverted to my old black-and-white thinking about food.

I thought I had to be the perfect eater in order to give nutritional advice to others. I never stopped to think that, if I allowed myself to be human, I could relate better to patients. I constantly kept myself in check during this time so I wouldn't go back to my old behaviors and harmful mindsets.

Eventually, I ended up in the field of eating disorders. I had arrived! This was my dream job, and I loved it.

People often asked me if working in this setting triggered disordered eating behavior for me. It definitely can trigger people in recovery. However, my work healed my relationship with food and increased my acceptance of my body.

My previous roles as a dietitian further perpetuated the diet mentality—the good and bad, the right and wrong. Working with eating disorders alongside other like-minded clinicians, I saw the dangers of diet culture every day and recognized the importance of mindfulness and the amorality of food (food is neither good nor bad).

My journey has not been easy. From time to time, I've had negative body-image days and have thought about food more than I care to do. I've compared and despaired and given in to maladaptive thoughts and beliefs. But for the most part, I walk in new freedom.

I would never have dreamed that, on my wedding night, I would stand before my husband, naked and unashamed. I could not have imagined how gracefully I would navigate body changes during pregnancy and continue to practice self-kindness on difficult days. I didn't think it possible to eat a slice of cake and move on with my life without wallowing in guilt. But it is possible, and I am living proof.

Our church often has a "real stories by real people" conversation on Sunday mornings before the message. During this time, a member of the church sits on the stage with our lead preacher and tells of a vulnerable time in their life, when they experienced unexpected joy through desperate dependence on Jesus. They may speak of loss, addiction, affairs, or any other difficult topic.

I always admire everyone's transparency when they share their stories of choosing healing over hiding. Our preacher often reminds us that we share our story to reveal His story. Our mess is our ministry. If I am not careful, I make much of me instead of making much of Him. But I am the most humble when I see where God has shown in up in my life.

At church, I've come across many people who have connected with me through different treatment facilities. None of these encounters were a coincidence. I've served alongside other women at church, co-leading a body-image group as part of our Recovery for Life ministry. I've seen women step out and share their struggles with food for the first time in their life. Many people from other churches have reached out to me and asked how to start a similar group in their communities. All along the way, I have seen God's hand at work.

While I was growing up in church, we sang a hymn called

Blessed Assurance. I grew up in the Church of Christ, where a song leader asked the congregation to turn to page 453 in the hymnal, and then he conducted from the stage. Now our family attends a church with a worship team and musical instruments. Gasp!

In this particular hymn, the chorus reads:

This is my story, this is my song
Praising my Savior all the day long
This is my story, this is my song
Praising my Savior all the day long

I'm learning that the workplace is our mission field. Each day, I have the opportunity to walk alongside individuals during some of the most vulnerable times of their lives. I have the chance to be a light to them as they do the hard work of recovery and silence the lies of diet culture. I'm learning that God can use my testimony to further His kingdom for His glory and not my own.

If you struggle with your body image or issues surrounding food, this book is for you. This book is my story revealing God's greater story and an invitation to you to walk in the same freedom I have. It is a call to be a critic of the media and to reject diet culture while seeking His truth about who we are and the image in which we were made.

I'm living proof that it's possible to walk in freedom from disordered eating and distorted beliefs. God can heal your relationship with food. I've seen Him do it with others, and He's done it for me. May you find strength to walk down this difficult path, knowing abundant life waits for you. This is my story. This is my song.

~ Two ~

UNWORTHY WEIGHT

At the time I'm writing this, Christian artist Lauren Daigel has recently released a new song titled, "You Say." The lyrics of her song talk about fighting thoughts that say she will never measure up. The song perfectly describes the constant battle in the mind of a person wrestling with disordered eating.

Eating disorders are tricky diseases. They prey upon the minds of their victims and make them believe the lie that they are not enough.

The lie slowly infiltrates the person's thoughts until they believe behaviors such as restricting, purging, or over-exercising will help them to measure up. They trick them into thinking the number on the scale or pant size can define their worth and identity.

Recently, I drove past a sign for a facility called Worthy Weight Loss. It makes me sad to see signs like this that reinforce the belief that our worth is tied to the number on a scale. Unfortunately, many individuals find their worth and identity, or lack thereof, in their weight and shape.

Others mask deeper-rooted issues as a simple weight problem. They believe their marriage would be better if they could lose weight. Or they think their career would work out if they could reach a certain number on the scale. It's easier to have a "weight problem" than a marriage or career problem.

The other day, I met with a patient who stated, "I have to get this weight off." I asked what would happen then. "My confidence would go up, and I'd have higher self-esteem."

We discussed the fact that a low weight doesn't always result in high self-esteem. I explained that many individuals in smaller bodies have poor self-esteem, while many individuals in larger-sized bodies have healthy self-esteem.

Self-esteem doesn't always depend upon body size. After digging deeper, we concluded that this self-acceptance issue was easier to label as a weight problem because that felt like something this person could control.

When individuals label deeper-rooted issues as weight problems, weight loss is never enough. They reach their goal weight and still have marriage issues, career struggles, and parenting battles.

Instead of realizing that the issue was never about the weight, they decide they have not yet lost enough. So they set their goal higher and continue on the journey of weight loss through restrictive dieting and other forms of self-punishment.

Just this morning, I met with a patient struggling in a romantic relationship. She believed her significant other's love for her was conditional upon her appearance. "I won't be loved if I don't have my dream body," she said. What an emotionally exhausting pursuit.

Some days she feels good in her own skin, deserving love. But most days, she experiences discomfort in her body, a sense of unworthiness, and body image dysmorphia (perceived defects or flaws in one's appearance). The emotional highs and lows leave her anxious, frustrated, and flat-out tired.

We talked about how our feelings are real, but not always reliable, and that she must remind herself of truth. When asked to come up with an alternative statement to her erroneous belief, she said, "My worth and identity are not found in my appearance."

Lauren Daigel's song goes on to say that in God she finds

her identity and worth. Not in a number on the scale. Not in a dress or pants size. Not in a kale salad with dressing on the side.

When we find our worth in Christ and who He says we are, we can walk in freedom and boldness as we work to heal our relationships with food and body. The chains of disordered eating can slowly break as we realize that our identity stands on a firm foundation, a solid rock.

I don't feel guilty when I order the extra serving of queso at my favorite Mexican restaurant or self-righteous when I have a kale salad for lunch. I don't find my worth in any of these things.

Neither do I sit in shame when my postpartum body doesn't fit into my pre-baby clothes. I don't feel morally superior when I choose to go for an evening run.

These events don't define my worth. My identity is in who God says I am and what He has done for me, not in anything I can do, and certainly not in any number.

You may think this all sounds great but wonder how to apply it to your life. Remember, as I stated earlier, our feelings are real but not always reliable. Therefore, we have to remind ourselves of truth.

Finding our true worth and identity is a slow process. It involves renewing our minds and altering our thoughts and belief system. It is a call to prayer, asking God to take away this burden of worrying about food and body to help you transform your mind and heart.

It's time to untangle our worth and our weight. Only then will we begin to experience true freedom from disordered eating. And then we can work to heal our relationship with food and practice body kindness while allowing the weight to fall naturally where it should.

Daigel's song ends with the final chorus describing who

God says she is, which is in stark contrast to how she feels, and ends with her declaring that she believes.

We will lose every time we let the number on the scale define our worth. Do you believe?

~ Three ~

WHAT THEY DON'T TEACH YOU
IN NUTRITION 101

I've been a mom for just shy of a year now. For almost twelve months, I've experienced the struggles of breastfeeding and postpartum body changes.

As I hurried out of my office last week, pumping supplies in hand, one of our dietary aides saw me and said, "Hey, Kristin, we're learning about nutrition during pregnancy and breast-feeding in my college nutrition class. I thought of you."

Cute. She gushed on and on about the curriculum and her new knowledge of breast milk and feeding a new baby. It all sounds sweet and magical. And it is, to some degree. However, before I can let her go on, I must interrupt and tell what nutrition during pregnancy and breastfeeding are really like. What they don't teach you in Nutrition 101.

They don't teach you that, when your milk first comes in, you wake up looking like a porn star with annoyingly perky, massive breasts, with which you have absolutely no idea what to do. All you know is they ache and leak, and you suddenly miss the size-A cup you took for granted all those years.

You also never hear that, after expressing breast milk, your boobs resemble those of a native woman on the cover of National Geographic. You know, the woman with no shirt on, ski-slope-like breasts, and a basket of fruit on her head.

If you're still not getting the image, visualize the power going out at your OB/GYN office and your breasts getting stuck in the mammogram machine for hours. They come out pancake-like, droopy, and inches farther from your face. You get the picture now.

Don't get me started on learning how to latch the baby. They forget to mention that this is similar to someone placing chip clips on your nipples and then telling you, "Good luck figuring out the rest."

Once, right after we came home from the hospital, my husband helped the baby to latch so I could feed our son while my husband ran an errand. I kid you not, the baby came unlatched, and neither my mom nor I could figure out how to get him back on.

We had to wait with sore nipples and a screaming baby until my husband returned to help. If the sales field doesn't work out for him, lactation consulting will.

You hear that nursing your baby is an intimate, special time between you and baby. However, I don't recall learning the baby may come at you like an angry bird at a worm. Not so intimate.

Professors lecture on the nutritional benefits of breast milk and the amazing way our bodies were created to produce just the right amounts of nutrients during each stage of development. But they don't tell you that the same hormone that plays a role in an orgasm is also responsible for milk letdown. This means that, late into the night, when your baby is fast asleep and you are trying to have four seconds of alone time with your husband, your nipples may alarm during sex. Then a less-than-attractive flow of milk will shower onto your husband and the bedsheets. I would have taken notes on that.

Breastfeeding is hard. Many well-meaning nutrition professors and professionals preach, "Breast is best." While I do believe breastfeeding benefits your baby, this message has resulted in unnecessary shame in women who aren't able to breastfeed.

I've sat with a mom who cried to the point of sickness because she wasn't producing enough breast milk to feed her baby. She was devastated to make the switch to formula, even though that ended up being best for her mental state. Plus, formula provided her son with the nutrition he lacked from the inadequate amount of breast milk.

When my friend decided to transition to formula after five months of breastfeeding, her OB/GYN asked, "Why did you stop? You could have lost more weight if you'd kept breastfeeding."

I was fortunate to have a large supply of breast milk from the beginning. We had no major feeding issues other than an enormous amount of pain during the first few weeks.

When our son was six months old, we moved to the country, which meant I had a much longer commute to work and was away from home longer during the day. Pumping during work has not been easy.

I share an office at the treatment center, so I borrow co-workers' offices when available. I have to schedule time to pump, clean my supplies, and find an area to store the milk. It is exhausting. As a result, I miss several pumps throughout the day, so my son takes a bottle or two of formula every day or every few days. At first, this discouraged me.

I felt a punch to the gut every time I saw the container of Similac in the pantry. It pained me to know he wasn't exclusively breastfed.

After a while, I began to wonder why this mattered so much to me. It wasn't an issue of whether or not my son would get adequate nourishment. On the contrary, he gets proper nutrition and is growing at just the right pace.

This wasn't a nutrition issue. It was a pride issue. I was tying my worth, or lack thereof, to my ability or inability to provide enough breast milk for my child.

I believe that "fed is best." "Fed" can come in many different forms. A dietitian once told me that "fed" is best, and so is a mentally stable mom. If your mental health suffers due to breastfeeding difficulties, it may not be worth it. Your baby needs you to take care of your mind so you can take care of the little one.

God continues to humble me in this area, as my breastfeeding journey is not over. I'd like to make it to twelve months of breastfeeding, but either way, my worth is not in such things.

I am a child of God. My worth is in Him and who He says I am. Not because of anything I have done, but because of all He has done.

Breastfeeding (or, for me, pumping) is hard. Everyone has a different story. Breastfeeding truly is a wonderful miracle that points us to the Creator.

However, mammas should remember that fed is best. Whatever way you have to do it, feeding the child is the priority. And please realize, dear mother—your worth is not tied to such things.

So whether you're poppin' out of your blouse or floppin' down to your waist, remember these words. And that is what they don't teach you in Nutrition 101.

~ Four ~

HOLY OR HOTTIE?

Our women's Bible study group is currently reading the book *Seamless*. In this study, author Angie Smith helps you to understand the Bible as one complete story. I've enjoyed navigating through the Old Testament and seeing how these stories are interwoven into the gospel. They still teach us today.

In the book of Joshua, Joshua leads the Israelites across the Jordan River to enter the Promised Land of Canaan. Many years passed since the exodus, and Moses has died, leaving Joshua as his successor. Joshua leads the Israelites into the land flowing with milk and honey. God instructs them to conquer the land and divide it between the twelve tribes of Israel.

In the book of Judges, the Promised Land has been divided, and God instructs each of the twelve tribes of Israel to conquer the land completely by driving out all the previous inhabitants. He told them to do this so the Canaanites, who worshipped false gods, wouldn't influence Israel to do the same.

However, the Israelites disobeyed God's command and did not drive out all the inhabitants of the land. As a result of the Canaanites' influence, God's people adopted many of their wicked practices. Eventually, they even asked for a king to rule over them.

In *Seamless*, Smith says, "The whole point for the Israelites was that God wanted to set them apart and make them different, but over and over again we see them wanting to be like everyone else."

God called the Israelites to be set apart for Him. But because of their disobedience, they fell into idol worship and became like those around them.

Merriam-Webster defines the word "holy" as "being set apart for the service of God." Like the Israelites, we are called to be holy and set apart. We are called to think differently, love differently, and act differently.

However, in the area of diet culture, we blend right in with the rest of the world. We give in to social pressures to look a certain way, eat a certain way, and follow the latest diet trends. We purchase the newest beauty products, try the latest diet fads, and pay a tremendous amount of money for memberships to the most upscale gyms.

We are just as dissatisfied with our bodies as the rest of the world. Like them, we search for the next best thing to make us feel better about ourselves. We may not ask for a literal king to rule over us, but we do bow down to the lordship of beauty, status, and the thin ideal.

We look to creation instead of the Creator to define our worth and identity, forgetting what God says about being image bearers of Christ.

It's easy to fall into the patterns of this world when we are constantly bombarded with messages saying we are not enough. Christians and non-Christians alike are victims of the toxic diet culture. Look no further than a television commercial, radio station, billboard, or magazine.

In a broken world desperate for something to define their worth and grasping for anything to give us identity, how do we as followers of Christ practice being holy and set apart for the service of God? I believe it starts with learning who we are in Him, deciding to believe His word is true and then living as if we believe it's true.

Let's start with some Bible passages that tell us who we are in Him and show us the importance (or lack of importance) of our appearance.

In Psalm 139:13-16, David proclaims, "You created my inmost being; you knit me together in my mother's womb. I praise you because I am fearfully and wonderfully made ... My frame was not hidden from you when I was made in the secret place, when I was woven together in the depths of the earth. Your eyes saw my unformed body." He goes on to say that God knew all the days of our lives, before any of them came to be.

If you grew up in the church as I did, you might skim over these words because you've heard them time and time again. However, in doing that, we miss out on these powerful statements.

The God of the universe knew my entire life from start to finish, before my parents even fathomed conceiving me, and He has loved me with an everlasting love. That truth can change lives.

In 1 Samuel 16, Samuel, a judge in Israel, goes to Bethlehem to visit a man named Jesse because the Lord is going to anoint one of his sons as the next king.

Samuel arrives, sees Jesse's son Eliab, and assumes he must be the one God chose to be king. But God tells Samuel, "'Do not consider his appearance or his height, for I have rejected him. The Lord does not look at the things people look at. People look at the outward appearance, but the Lord looks at the heart'" (verse 7).

Isaiah 53:2 says, "He had no beauty or majesty to attract us to him, nothing in his appearance that we should desire him." This verse refers to the coming Messiah.

So we read that God created us and knows us intimately. We also know God values our hearts more than our appearance.

Based on what God's Word says about who we are, we have

a decision to make. Are we going to believe it or not?

When I get frustrated and confused and don't understand God, I remind myself that I am not made to understand all His plans and all His ways. I come back to the same question time and time again. Do I believe Him, or do I not? I've concluded that I can't believe part of His Word without believing all of it.

So I either believe it's true or I don't. I've decided that I believe His Word is true. Hebrews 4:12 says that the word of God is alive and active and sharper than any double-edged sword.

If I know who God's Word says I am, and I believe it's true, then I must live as though I believe it's true. In the areas of food and body, I must act in a way that aligns with my belief: my worth and identity are in Christ alone.

I do not find my worth in my weight, dress size, workout plan, or the number of calories I've eaten. I do not bow down to the idol of the thin ideal. I make health important but not ultimate. I honor God with my body, treating it as a temple of the Holy Spirit. I practice self-care through balanced eating and mindful movement, and I refrain from fat shaming or diet talk.

Are you willing to be holy and set apart for God's service? Do you know what God's word says about who you are in Him? Do you believe it's true? If so, are you willing to let it change your life? Because I promise you, if we genuinely believe this stuff, it will change our lives.

Remember, this is not a diet book. It is not a self-help book on weight loss, balanced eating, or healthy cooking. You can find lots of resources on those topics, but this is not one of them.

The purpose of this book is to challenge you to examine yourself and determine how to define your worth and identity. This book specifically focuses on areas relating to food, body image, and diet culture. It's an invitation to view these topics through a faith-based lens.

I hope you will receive helpful tips and tricks along the way, so you can make peace with food and practice mindful eating. But my ultimate goal is for you to close the last chapter of this book and rededicate your life to God, placing your worth on the firm foundation of His love, and experiencing the breaking of chains in the area of disordered eating. Here's to continuing on our journey!

~ Five ~

#CleanEating

I am talented at many things. Technology is not one of them. I think I may have been born in the wrong era because I often feel as if I shouldn't be living among this tech-savvy generation.

When Facebook Live became a thing, I said to my husband, "Oh, look, Tiffany is on live, selling clothes." He waved and said, "Hey, Tiff!" Bless his heart. We were meant for each other. I had to break it to him that this was not the same thing as Facetime, and Tiffany couldn't see or hear us.

When we were first engaged, I took a picture of my ring and posted it to my Facebook page. But it accidentally posted under my ex-boyfriend's account because somehow his account was still set to my Facebook app. As you can imagine, I started receiving texts from friends asking me why my ex was posting the news of my engagement. My now-husband and I scrambled to figure out how to remove the post.

I recently joined Instagram (I know, I'm behind the times) and noticed that I immediately gained followers after creating my account. I had to ask my friend what exactly it was they were following since I had not yet figured out how to post anything.

I quickly discovered that messages centering around food and body are everywhere on Instagram.

With the rise in social media through Facebook, Instagram, and Pinterest comes an increase in comparison, competition, and false advertising. This rise can lead to feelings of inadequacy, discontentment, and worthlessness.

How crazy that something taking up so much of our time leaves us feeling worse about ourselves. How bizarre that a pastime meant to create connectedness leaves us feeling disconnected and discontented.

With this increase in social media comes the growth of trendy diets, food photography, pill-pushing with pyramid schemes, nutritional supplements, and never-ending selfies at the gym. We see the detoxes, the cleanses, and the cute new workout attire (without the gym sweat).

We all know this, yet no one embraces it. People post only what they want you to see. The life they want you to think they live.

They post pictures of a balanced meal in an immaculate kitchen with no trace of crumbs or mail on the dinner table. Their hashtags: #cleaneating, #detox, #cleanse, #healthy.

How come no one ever posts #atetoomanychipsandsalsa, #bloated, #thankfulforstretchypants? This is real life. This is what happens to all of us at some point, not because we are gluttons, but because we are human.

Yet this part of the story gets left out, leaving us to scroll through our newsfeeds, assuming we're the only person in the world ever to feel slightly out of control or off balance. As a result, we have feelings of guilt and shame that keep us in vicious diet cycles and patterns of self-loathing.

The problem with this clean-eating movement is that it makes eating a moral situation. It categorizes food as good or bad, leaving me to believe that if I ate something bad, I am now bad. If my plate does not hold freshly picked produce or resemble something from a Top Chef episode, I feel inadequate. If I'm not eating clean, then I feel dirty, bad, and sinful.

I work with patients all the time to help them see that not all food is nutritionally equal, but it should be emotionally equal so I can have an apple without feeling self-righteous, and I can have a brownie without feeling guilty or shameful.

Jesus himself declared all foods clean in Mathew 15:11 by saying that what goes into someone's mouth does not defile them, but what comes out of their mouth defiles them.

When we think eating bad food is the problem, we are left to believe eating clean food (dieting) is the solution. We are stuck in the diet cycle of restricting, breaking food rules, and overeating due to the "What the heck?" mentality we get when we've blown the diet. Then our feelings of guilt and shame trigger further restriction or continuous dieting. Sound exhausting? It is.

Why don't we try being more real and transparent? If we want to post the perfect plate, why don't we also post the delicious ice cream cone we had on Friday night after filling our bellies at the local Mexican restaurant?

Why don't we honor our hunger as well as our fullness and enjoy the pleasures of eating a variety of foods and food groups? Eat a well-balanced, homemade meal at the dinner table some nights, but at other times, have a frozen pizza in front of the television.

We should challenge the status quo that has turned food into a moral situation—a right and wrong, a black and white, a good and bad. This leaves us with a hunger for something more than food.

I challenge you to log off, disconnect, and nourish yourself with food, family, friends, and health. With balance, honesty, self-care, and compassion. Connect with the real world and with the things that matter. A healthy relationship with food will trump the perfect Instagram filter every time. Only then will you taste a life of #progressoverperfection, #healthybodyimage, and #havemycakeandeatittoo.

The life I wish for you is for you to be free from the chains of comparison, self-criticism, and disordered eating. Live a life like a box of chocolates. Log off, disconnect, and live.

~ Six ~

JESUS ATE CARBS

"I am the bread of life. Whoever comes to me will never go hungry, and whoever believes in me will never be thirsty" (John 6:35).

Have you ever seen those t-shirts that say, "Jesus drank wine"? Sometimes I'm not sure how I feel about those shirts because I think some people use that as an excuse to get drunk, or they take His wine drinking out of context.

But sometimes I think they're cute, and I want to add, "Jesus ate carbs."

If you read through the Bible, you will find a multitude of food and drink analogies. John 4:4-30 tells the story of the woman at the well.

Jesus is in Samaria and sits near a well. About that time, a Samaritan woman comes to draw water. If you look at the context of this story, this woman is an outcast. Being a Samaritan, she is looked down upon by the Jews. We later learn she is also a prostitute.

The story says she approached the well around noon, the hottest time of the day. Her timing might mean she purposely came when other women would not be present, and she would be left alone.

Jesus asks this woman for a drink. His question quickly leads to a much deeper discussion. He tells her He can offer living water, and in verses 13-14, He says, "Everyone who drinks this water will be thirsty again, but whoever drinks the water I give them will never thirst. Indeed, the water I give them will become in them a spring of water welling up to eternal life." He is the living water He speaks of.

In John 6:35, Jesus refers to Himself as the bread of life. In verses 49-51, He says, "Your ancestors ate the manna in the wilderness, yet they died. But here is the bread that comes down from heaven, which anyone may eat and not die. I am the living bread that came down from heaven. Whoever eats this bread will live forever. This bread is my flesh, which I will give for the life of the world."

He is both living water and the bread of life.

Another interesting passage on the topic of bread is in Exodus 16:4. In it, God promised the Israelites that He would rain down bread from heaven as they wandered in the wilderness before entering the Promised Land.

This bread was their daily provision. When the people gathered more than a day's worth, it grew maggots and began to smell.

The Israelites were to trust God daily for what they needed. They had no plan for the future. They were to trust God one day at a time.

So again, Jesus is living water and the bread of life, and He provides our daily bread. In the Lord's Prayer, He instructed us to pray for, but not worry about, this daily bread. We are to focus on the needs at hand one day at a time.

He is the living water and the bread of life, and He provides our daily bread.

And I like to think He probably ate carbs.

Seven

STARS AND DOTS

You Are Special by Max Lucado is my all-time favorite children's book. I love to give it at baby showers. In this book, Punchinello was a Wemmick, a small wooden person. He lived with other Wemmicks made by Eli, the woodworker. The Wemmicks walked through the village daily, giving each other stickers. Stars were the most prized. If a Wemmick received a star, this meant he possessed something valuable in the sight of all the other villagers. Perhaps they were beautiful or talented or creative. Each of these assets earned them a star.

Other Wemmicks, like Punchinello, received dots, which represented ordinary, subpar, or misfit Wemmicks. Punchinello walked throughout the village, head downcast, wearing his dots.

One day he met another Wemmick named Lucia. Punchinello felt drawn to Lucia, for she did not have any stars or dots on her. When Punchinello inquired about her lack of stickers, Lucia said she had none because she visited Eli the woodcarver daily.

One day, Punchinello went to visit Eli himself. Eli said, "I don't care what other Wemmicks think. All that matters is what I think. And I think you are pretty special."

Surprised by this comment, Punchinello went on to ask Eli why stickers do not stay on Lucia. He replied, "Because she has decided that what I think is more important than what they think. The stickers only stick if you let them."

You're probably thinking that there is no need for you to go out and purchase this book now that I've told you the main plot.

However, I'll save the ending as a surprise. You'll have to read it to find out what happens!

You also might wonder if you are still reading a book about not finding your worth and identity in your weight. Maybe you flipped back to the front cover to make sure you hadn't somehow ended up in a children's devotional. Keep tracking with me.

I think we are a lot like Wemmicks. We walk around and let people stick dots on us. And if we are honest with ourselves, we also stick ourselves with dots.

The diet industry is a sixty-billion-dollar industry, and it profits from people's negative self-image and desire to change their bodies. They earn money by making us feel bad about ourselves, then convincing us that something about us is broken, and they have the magic ingredient to "fix" us.

Every time we give in to a commercial, buy a weight-loss product, or stand on the scale in an attempt to change ourselves, the industry sticks a dot on us. And because we've lived and thought this way far too long, we forget that we can alter our thoughts, challenge our beliefs, and renew our minds.

So we carry on because, although it's painful, it's sometimes the easiest route. And we go along wearing our dots. However, our feelings are real but not necessarily reliable.

We have to remind ourselves of the truth: we are all unworthy. That's the whole point of the gospel. Jesus came to die because we could not save ourselves.

He calls us worthy, not because of anything we have done, but because of what He did on the cross. The question is: do we believe Him? Are we willing to let Him place a star on us while the dot falls to the ground?

As much as I hate to admit it, we cannot escape diet culture. It's all around us. Some of us don't even have to go outside our homes to feel its influence. Turn on your television, turn up your radio, or scroll through your newsfeed. The diet culture is every-where.

Will you listen to it? Will you internalize the lies and allow them to place dots on you? Or will you turn to the Maker and choose God's truth over man's opinion? Will you keep your focus on the Creator and open His Word to see what He says about you? Will you believe He knows the number of hairs on your head and knew all the days of your life before one of them came to be?

You must decide who to listen to—the media or the Maker, creation or the Creator, Wemmicks or the Woodcarver. I hope that, like Lucia, you will decide that God's opinion matters more than others'. And before you know it, a dot just might fall off.

~ Eight ~

BRONZE SNAKES

Do you not know that your bodies are temples of the Holy Spirit, who is in you, whom you have received from God? You are not your own; you were bought at a price. Therefore honor God with your bodies (1 Corinthians 6:19-20).

The Old Testament contains countless records of times when the Israelites, God's chosen people, abandoned the one true God and fell into idolatry.

After the reign of King Solomon, the kingdom was divided into the Northern Kingdom (Israel) and the Southern Kingdom (Judah). Israel had fallen and was taken into exile. Judah would follow suit if they refused to turn from their evil ways.

Hezekiah became king of Judah and, according to 2 Kings 18:3, "he did what was right in the eyes of the Lord." King Hezekiah worked to destroy all forms of idol worship and "broke into pieces the bronze snake Moses had made, for up to that time the Israelites had been burning incense to it" (verse 4).

In the book of Numbers, we read that Moses created the snake to cure the Israelites from poisonous snakebites. God wanted to display His power as well as His presence among His people.

What was meant to point Israel back to their Creator had become an object of pagan worship. We should be careful that our instruments of worship do not become the very things we worship.

When it comes to our bodies, good health should encourage

us to worship the Creator. What happens, however, when we start to worship the created? What happens when we take something good and make it ultimate?

According to the National Eating Disorder Association, the term orthorexia means an obsession with proper or "healthful" eating. Though not yet included in the Diagnostic and Statistical Manual of Mental Disorders at the time of this writing, people with orthorexia become fixated on so-called healthy eating to the point that they damage their own well-being.

What if today's bronze snakes are clean eating, detox diets, and fitness challenges? What if our culture has transitioned from thanking God for the food on our table to worshipping it? What if we have placed our hope in our pants' size and let a number on the scale define our worth?

When we take a good thing, such as health, and make it ultimate, we trade the Creator for the created, the Giver for the gift, and the Potter for the clay. Not only is this sinful, but it also leaves us feeling discouraged, exhausted, and disappointed time and time again.

Psalm 135:15-18 says,

The idols of the nations are silver and gold, made by human hands. They have mouths, but cannot speak, eyes, but cannot see. They have ears, but cannot hear, nor is there breath in their mouths. Those who make them will be like them, and so will all who trust in them.

As the saying goes, you are what you eat. I believe we live in a generation that feels hopeless and unworthy, a generation confused about their identity, willing to grasp at anything in order to find purpose and meaning in life.

I believe we live in a culture that lets their actions define who they are instead of letting who they are define what they do.

Isaiah 44:9 says, "All who make idols are nothing, and the things they treasure are worthless."

Do you think that when you get to the gates of heaven, God will ask if you got in all 10,000 steps on your Fit Bit each day on earth? Do you think He'll want an account of each clean-eating recipe on your Pinterest board, along with an Instagram photo of the finished product?

This idea convicts me time and time again. For instance, I feel guilty when I invest more time into creating my weekly grocery list than I do in the lives of people around me. Or when I am more concerned with missing a workout than a morning quiet time.

Many professionals preach that Americans are dealing with a health issue. I believe we are dealing with a heart issue.

The prophet Jeremiah warned the people about their idolatry and urged them to repent. He prophesied about God's judgment and condemned Judah for its sins. "I will pronounce my judgments on my people because of their wickedness in forsaking me, in burning incense to other gods and in worshipping what their hands have made" (Jeremiah 1:16).

Judah had placed its trust in what their hands had made. They placed their hope in the created instead of the Creator.

What happens when we do the same with our health? What happens when we place our hope and trust in our diet and exercise? What happens when we develop an incurable illness, a tragic and unexpected cancer diagnosis?

A close friend in our home group received a cancer diagnosis a few years ago. What began as a little stomachache soon became much more. For months and months, she visited doctors, eliminated certain food groups due to a false food allergy diagnosis, and dealt with severe gastrointestinal pains.

One day, her husband called and told us she couldn't keep anything down, so he was taking her to the ER. The doctors diagnosed her with a small bowel obstruction from a tumor. She had surgery to remove the tumor along with a portion of her intestines. The tumor tested positive for cancer.

That moment devastated my friend and her husband. How could a twenty-five-year-old healthy woman with a balanced diet and active lifestyle get a cancer diagnosis?

Walking through that dark time with our friends helped me to understand further that I cannot place my hope in my health. Health is important and a blessing to be grateful for, but it will never be a solid rock to stand on. It is sinking sand, just like all the other false idols we place our trust in: success, money, material possessions. All can become bronze snakes or golden calves if we are not careful.

Jeremiah 2:13 says, "'My people have committed two sins: They have forsaken me, the spring of living water, and have dug their own cisterns, broken cisterns that cannot hold water.'"

A cistern is a tank or pit that stores rainwater, especially one supplying taps or a toilet. Now compare that to a spring of living water: cold, refreshing, quenching our thirsty souls. And to think we would choose toilet water over this.

We live in a culture that thirsts for worth and identity, value and belonging. But we will never find these things on a plate of kale or through a Lifetime Fitness membership. We've taken something good and made it ultimate. We've worshipped the creation instead of the Creator.

Let us fix our eyes on Jesus and put Him back in His rightful place in our hearts. Let us be wary of placing our hope in our health. May we rest in being who God says we are instead of pursuing our identity in what we have eaten or the number of calories we have burned. Let us be a generation that detoxes, not from food, but from the poisonous ideas of diet culture and the lies that tell us our value is in a number.

Let us be a generation that does not worship the idols of health, weight, and fitness. All these good things, if made ultimate in our hearts, are nothing more than ugly bronze snakes.

~ Nine ~

THE TABLE

If your kitchen table is anything like mine, it has many functions. We use it as a desk by holding mail, bills, invitations, and advertisements. It is a landing place for a heavy purse and leather briefcase at the end of a long workday.

The kitchen chairs act as clotheslines for freshly washed linens that cannot be placed in the dryer. This turns awkward when you have to snatch clean panties from the kitchen chairs as dinner guests arrive.

Dinnertime in our house often involves pushing all our belongings to one side of the table to clear space for our plates. I don't know why, but having things on the kitchen table has always been a pet peeve of mine. I want the table to be a welcoming place for someone to come and rest and receive nourishment at any given time, not a crowded fast-food restaurant where the workers rush to give the table a swipe before anyone can be seated.

Recently, my husband and I went shopping for a dining room table. We wanted something big, a table that could seat lots of friends and family. We walked around the furniture store, discussing options and comparing our preferences.

He liked strong and sturdy wooden chairs with a matching distressed bench. I preferred soft, warm cloth chairs that invite someone to stay for deep conversation and laughs long after the meal is over.

We compromised and left that day with a long wooden distressed table, five strong and sturdy wooden chairs, a bench, and two soft, warm cloth chairs for the ends. We arrived home and arranged everything perfectly. Then we added a deep, oval wooden centerpiece holding dark-green moss balls and six straw placemats.

Since that time, we've had small dinners for two with homemade pizza and a bottle of wine. We've hosted family for Mother's Day with roast beef, potatoes, and all the fixings, and we've had friends over on summer nights to grill and then catch up around the table.

We've celebrated engagements, cried over losses, caught up with old friends, discussed Jesus and finances with mentors, laughed over inside jokes, and swapped marriage stories all around the table.

In her book *Bread and Wine*, Shauna Niequist talks about the importance of gathering loved ones around your table. She says, "Learn, little by little, meal by meal, to feed yourself and the people you love because food is one of the ways we love each other and the table is one of the most sacred places that we gather."

In today's diet culture, we've lost the importance of gathering around the table. We are so controlled by rigid food rules and busy schedules that we no longer take time to nourish ourselves and loved ones and to enjoy the satisfaction of a home-cooked meal. In fact, sometimes we don't even believe we deserve satisfaction from eating.

I'm intrigued by places like France, where people sit at cafes for hours, eating rich foods and enjoying meaningful conversation. There the server doesn't breathe down your neck, eager to give you your check so the next party can sit at your table. It's a place where customers don't walk away feeling guilty after their meal but are simply grateful for the pleasure of eating.

Did you know that the United States is one of the only

countries whose dietary guidelines don't list anything about the enjoyment of eating and the pleasure we should find in food?

I wonder if we are so busy obsessing over our "obesity epidemic" that we miss out on the most important part. We live in fear that, if we enjoy our food, we might not be able to stop eating, and we might gain weight. So we stick to restrictive diets or fast, convenient meals and go about our lives.

What if we took time to clear off our tables and clear out our minds? What if we slowed down, poured a glass of wine, and gathered our ingredients for a new recipe while Frank Sinatra played on Pandora in the background?

What if we invited people into our less-than-perfect homes and into our real lives, sharing a meal with them? What if we learned what it meant to nourish and care for our bodies properly while finding satisfaction in eating?

For centuries, the table has been an important place. Jesus gathered His twelve disciples around the table at the Last Supper, symbolically broke the bread and sipped the wine, prophetically predicting His body broken and His blood poured out as a sacrificial offering for our sins.

Are you tired of punishing yourself through restrictive diets and rigid eating rules? Do you tirelessly keep up with the latest health trend and experience a decreased quality of life because of it? Are you worn down, depressed, and hungry for more than food can offer?

Gather around the table.

~ Ten ~

SUMMERTIME, SNOW CONES, AND SIZE ACCEPTANCE

This past weekend, my eighteen-month-old nephew came to visit. Hayden is a joy to be around. He is funny and smart and tenderhearted, and he has a contagious laugh, a smile that melts your heart, and big, ocean-blue eyes. He loves to play with his John Deere dump truck, blow bubbles in the backyard, throw the ball for his dog, Clover, and press any and every button or light he can get his hands on.

Because he is the first grandchild of the family, my parents have gone all out since the day he was born. My mom has new toys and clothes waiting for him every time he comes to visit, and my dad plans to take him camping on our family land. My parents flood Hayden with new forms of entertainment every time he's in town. This past weekend was no different.

Their backyard looked like a theme park, complete with a blow-up elephant pool with a slide and inflatable palm tree, a new sandbox with big buckets and colorful shovels, a blue rocking horse, and a snow-cone maker with assorted colors and flavors from which to choose.

When I arrived at my parents' house after work one evening, I found Hayden running around the backyard, his turquoise swim trunks on, a big, bright smile on his face, and cherry-red snow-cone juice running down his chin and across his belly.

As a toddler, Hayden loves to feed himself, which means that sometimes food makes it into his mouth, and sometimes it doesn't. But Hayden didn't mind that day. He just dipped his little spoon into his icy-cold snow cone and pulled out a heaping mound of cherry-flavored ice. He laughed as most of it dribbled down his face.

Then, cherry-stained from the tip of his nose to the bottom of his belly button, Hayden proceeded to splash around in his pool, build sandcastles, and enjoy the summer day.

There's something intriguing about the way toddlers freely play and enjoy their bodies. Their curiosity starts in infancy when they explore their toes, soft, bulging belly, and wiggly fingers. Then they discover what a newly discovered body part can do and how it works. They laugh when they learn the joy of clapping their hands and patting their belly.

Toddlers are untainted by a diet culture and a cruel world that makes money by brainwashing people to hate their bodies and distrust their hunger signals. They don't know a world where we hide shame behind a swimsuit cover-up and use hashtags to discuss beach bodies and summer-ready diets.

As adults, we dread shopping for a bathing suit and worry about burning off the calories we ate at a summer cookout. Most of us wouldn't be caught dead running around in swim trunks with cherry-red snow cone dripping down our bellies.

Children have a lot to tell us about eating, body trust, and size acceptance. They teach us we can learn something new about ourselves each day and be thankful for a healthy and able body. They also show us that the foundational component of proper nutrition and a healthy relationship with food is learning how to accept and embrace our current bodies versus striving for the thin ideal.

Children model the importance of not letting guilt or shame keep us from living an abundant life and enjoying time with loved ones this summer. They don't put their lives on hold until they reach a goal weight.

When Hayden took a bath that night, he patted his belly like a drum and laughed at the funny noise it made. He kicked his feet and tried to snap his fingers like he'd seen his Pawpaw doing earlier in the evening.

Hayden may not always love every little detail about his body. He may grow up and notice flaws or imperfections. He might have challenges to face. But this past weekend, Hayden accepted his body and enjoyed his summer to the fullest. Sandbox, swimming pool, cherry-red-stained belly, and all.

~ Eleven ~

WHY I NO LONGER FEAR HUNGER

This week marked twenty weeks into my first pregnancy. I am halfway to meeting my precious baby boy. Pregnancy has been interesting so far, with wide ranges of emotions, weird sleeping positions, frequent trips to the bathroom, and an ever-changing body (and I still have twenty weeks to go).

When a woman announces she's expecting, her body suddenly becomes fair game for discussing and critiquing. A colleague told my friend she looked as if she would have her baby any day, although her due date was months away. My sister's friend recently heard that she didn't look far enough along, based on her due date.

Recently my co-worker said, "You look as if you went on break for Thanksgiving and came back pregnant." A family friend said, "You must be having a boy because of the way you're carrying him."

The best was yesterday evening when I was leaving work, and a man on the elevator exclaimed, "Baby bump!" The women in the elevator looked uncomfortable. One said, "I wasn't going to say anything." Apparently some men don't know the rule: even if a woman is nine months pregnant and in labor, you never assume she is having a baby unless she tells you. I laughed and told the man he was right—my bump was a baby.

As we got off the elevator, I joked with him, saying, "I should have said, 'Nope! Just finished dinner!'" He laughed in return and said how embarrassed he would have been. The other women chuckled. They knew this assumption could have gone so wrong.

On the other hand, I enjoyed a comment from the Salvation Army volunteer ringing her bell outside Hobby Lobby. "You're glowing!" I'm not sure if the glow was from my pregnancy or the 50-percent-off discount, but I'll take it.

The most precious comments come from friends and family who speak directly to my baby. It takes the focus off my body and places the attention on this little man in the womb.

I loved hearing my mother-in-law whisper, "GiGi loves you!" and my mother crooning, "You're going to love playing with your big cousin Hayden." My husband talks to my belly every night. He has said some of the most meaningful and hilarious things.

What amazes me even more are the comments I hear regarding eating. "You're eating for two now." "I bet you appreciated Thanksgiving this year since you have the excuse of being pregnant. Enjoy it now while you can."

It's as if some foods are suddenly off limits once you are no longer pregnant. The clock strikes twelve, and you have to go back to being a "good" eater.

From a nutrition standpoint, I know the old concept of eating for two is a myth, and that women typically need only about 300-500 additional calories in the second and third trimester of pregnancy. This addition only amounts to half a peanut butter sandwich and eight ounces of milk. Hardly a feast.

The people who express these notions are well-meaning and never intentionally harmful. But these comments can send the unspoken message that we should enjoy food only under certain circumstances and that we should indulge in foods we love only during special times in our lives.

I've met with many patients who tell me they're scared of experiencing hunger. Some may constantly eat throughout the day to avoid feeling the slightest hunger pang. Others restrict to the point of dulling all physical sensations, such as a stomach growl.

The main reason for this, they report, is a common fear of being out of control with their eating. They worry that, if they feel hungry, they might eat and then be unable to stop. They may have trouble differentiating between physical and emotional hunger and may also eat for unrelated reasons.

They view their body as the enemy instead of an ally. They never stop to think that their body might be trying to tell them something worth stopping and listening to.

Throughout my pregnancy, I've followed a phone app called The Bump. Each week, I receive updates about the size and development of my growing baby and changes to expect in my body.

Around weeks nineteen and twenty, new moms are told to expect leg cramps, heartburn/indigestion, and shortness of breath. (Oh, yay.) We are also advised to expect an increase in hunger during this time. The baby grows at a much more rapid pace at this stage, creating increased nutritional needs for both mom and baby.

Up until this point, I haven't experienced many changes in my hunger or eating patterns. I had occasional food aversions in the first trimester (cooked vegetables—gross!). I still haven't experienced the stereotypical desire for ice cream and a pickle or an unquenchable thirst for anything in particular, other than red wine. (Sparkling water will do for now.)

This week, as I enter into my twentieth week of pregnancy, I feel hungrier. In the past, when I struggled with eating and body-image issues, hunger scared me as it scares my patients today. I feared that if I ate every time I was hungry, I would gain weight and feel off-balance somehow. I didn't believe I could trust my own body or that it somehow innately knew what it was doing. I thought I needed to be the one in control.

Little did I know that ignoring hunger cues is like pulling back a rubber band. You can pull back only so far until it eventually flies across the room, leading to out-of-control eating.

For me, ignoring hunger typically led to overeating later in the day. Other times, it led to inappropriate dietary restrictions that sent me down the path of an eating disorder.

Through my experience of making peace with food, becoming an intuitive eater, and my work as a dietitian specializing in the treatment of eating disorders, I learned that our bodies are amazing tools. They help us navigate hunger, fullness, balance, and enjoyment if we allow them to.

We are fearfully and wonderfully made and can trust our bodies to know exactly what they are doing and precisely what we need. Just as my body knows how to grow and nourish a child in the womb for nine months, my body also knows when I need an extra burst of energy via food.

Instead of viewing my body as an enemy or hunger as something to fear, I now see them as guides, leading me through the process of mindful eating. I know that if I feel my stomach growl and ignore the sensation by continuing to work and not stopping to eat, I could become fatigued, irritable, and even lightheaded. Not eating could also trigger me to overeat later in the day.

I now know that, when my body sends hunger cues, I must listen and respect them. I can trust that fullness cues will help me to eat just the amount my body needs. I know that at times I'll overeat simply because the food tastes good. Or I might unconsciously use food to deal with an unmet emotional need, boredom, or fatigue.

At other times, I may eat too little because I'm rushed for

time or don't have available food. All in all, I can trust my body. It knows how to digest food, absorb nutrients, and store energy. It works in perfect balance, keeping me in a place of homeostasis.

This pregnancy journey has been full of emotional ups and downs and learning curves along the way. It's been nothing short of a miracle, and I'm grateful to my body for knowing exactly how to provide for and protect my precious unborn son.

I'm learning that hunger is nothing to be feared but rather something to be embraced. Our bodies have something to teach us about eating, health, pleasure, and creation if we let them.

~ Twelve ~

PREPARE FOR TAKEOFF

I have an irrational fear of flying. I hate the drop in my stomach during turbulence. I always have bad flashbacks of vomiting on the Judge Roy Scream at Six Flags. I see the ocean beneath me and just know the plane will soon turn into a life raft with hungry sharks waiting to reenact the Jaws movies. I tremble when I see suspicious-looking passengers. Did they somehow bypass the TSA line at the airport?

I've seen kid passengers who are more courageous than I am. I beg my husband to upgrade his boarding pass to make sure we can sit together. Then I nearly break his arm by using it as a stress ball as the plane ascends into the air.

It's an irrational fear. I know the facts. Millions of planes fly daily and make it to their destination safely. I'm more likely to experience danger while driving on the highway than while flying on a plane.

Part of the reason I'm afraid of flying is that I don't do it often. I fly maybe once a year or every few years. Therefore, each flight is a scary experience for me.

A businessman who travels for work frequently, however, likely has little to no fear of flying, because he does it all the time. He's used to it. It has become a habit. But unless I face my fear and fly, I will never reach my destination.

This fear of flying is similar to recovering from disordered eating. Certain foods have been put off limits due to rigid eating rules or a strict diet mentality. They appear unsafe and even scary. We fear gaining weight or losing control if we do eat them. This fear might consume our thoughts and increase our anxiety.

You may have told yourself, "You shouldn't have that," or "That is bad," or "You can have this only if you work out afterward."

Intuitive eaters, on the other hand, can eat what they want and then continue their day without thinking about it anymore. Intuitive eaters eat when they are hungry and stop when they are full. They trust their body's internal cues, find satisfaction in eating, and cope with emotions without using food. Sounds almost too good to be true, doesn't it?

If some people can eat this way, why do others find it challenging to face their fears of certain foods?

It's the same as the traveling businessman. He is better able to manage his fears because he flies frequently. He's used to flying, and it has become a habit for him. He's experienced safe takeoffs and landings.

Intuitive eaters are used to experiencing freedom in food choices. They are familiar with the idea of eating when they are hungry, and they recognize and honor fullness cues. No foods are off limits. All foods are safe and readily available.

The intuitive eater can eat half of their favorite dish and pass up the other half when they are satisfied, knowing that when they are hungry again, they can eat again. Because no foods are off limits, food loses its power. Now the power lies within the eater to make their own food choices.

This way of eating becomes a habit for the intuitive eater. They aren't weighed down by endless food rules and confusing emotions.

A dietitian friend once told me the story of the red truck. This story has stuck with me for years, and I have passed it down to numerous patients and colleagues.

It goes like this: A bunch of kids is sitting in a playroom, surrounded by dozens of toys. The babysitter announces, "I'll be right back. Play with anything you want to in this room, except for the red truck. It is off limits." As soon as she leaves, the kids dash for the red truck.

Remember, they are in a room full of toys. However, they want the red truck simply because it is forbidden. Do you know who doesn't want the red truck? The kid who has this exact toy at home. He can take it or leave it. It's no big deal to him because it is part of his regular, everyday life.

Food is no different for us. The dieters eventually rush to the off-limit foods (triggering overeating and then another diet), and the intuitive eaters can take it or leave it—no big deal.

I often tell my patients that explaining the concept of intuitive eating to a chronic dieter is much like trying to tell someone what it would be like to live underwater. It sounds great, but you haven't experienced it for yourself. It has never been a reality for you, so the idea is exciting, scary, and strange at the same time.

How then do we work toward becoming an intuitive eater? We face our fears in the same way we conquer our fear of flying—we get on the plane and prepare for takeoff.

A painted quote by an unknown author hangs on a wall at the eating disorder treatment facility where I used to work. It says, "Sometimes the fear will not go away, so you will just have to do it afraid."

I have a love-hate relationship with this quote. I love it because it's true. Sometimes the fear doesn't go away. Sometimes God doesn't equip us with courage until we are in the throes of the thing that scares us. But we learn and grow when we face our fears.

But I also hate this quote because who wants to face their

fears afraid? I'd love to hear that the fear would just disappear, and I'd be brave. But that isn't real life, and that's not where recovery happens or where faith is strengthened.

This idea of facing food fears may look different for everyone. One size doesn't fit all. It might mean making a list of all your fear foods. These are the foods you once liked but are now afraid to eat due to fear of gaining weight or losing control of your eating.

It may look like slowly adding these foods into your meal plan, safely and structured, while working to manage your anxiety and fear of these foods. In time, the fear decreases, and eating normalizes. We call this exposure-response prevention.

Exposure-response prevention is a form of therapy in which the therapist exposes the patient to certain triggers that elicit anxiety, followed by disordered behavior. Response prevention helps the individual not to act upon urges to engage in the disordered behaviors when triggered. This treatment is done under the guidance of a therapist or registered dietitian, and, in time, the individual can better manage the anxiety surrounding the triggers.

For a particular patient of mine, this looked like going to Dunkin Donuts and ordering just one donut to eat there. You see, this patient associated Dunkin Donuts with binging. Donuts triggered binging for him. He felt out of control every time he ate them. He binged because he believed this would be his last time to eat donuts.

One day, under the supervision of his psychologist, he went to Dunkin Donuts. He ordered one donut, sat down, and ate it mindfully while paying attention to his environment.

He noticed other people eating their donuts and enjoying the company of friends. As he took the first bite of his donut, he noted that flakes of sugar sprinkled down his shirt. He finished his donut, gathered his things, and then left to process this experience with his therapist.

Practicing these types of experiments over time led him to take control over the food and place it in his own hands. Over time, eating one to two donuts at Dunkin Donuts became a habit. He got used to it. Eating donuts no longer triggered overeating because he knew that when he was hungry for donuts again, he could always go back. He had his cake—or donut—and ate it too.

Our feelings are real but not necessarily reliable. Although I may feel fat or out of control after eating a particular food, I may not be fat or out of control. In those moments of intense feelings, I have to remind myself of truth.

When you feel fearful, it may help to remind yourself of the facts. Just as I know millions of planes take off daily and make it to their destination safely, I know that 3,500 calories create one pound of fat, making it highly unlikely that one particular food item would cause weight gain.

A patient recently came into my office, convinced that adding croutons to her salad over the weekend had caused her to gain weight. I reminded her that she had to eat 3,500 calories worth of croutons on her salad in order to gain one pound. She was surprised at this and quickly reported that she knew she had not eaten that many croutons.

After reviewing the facts, she felt more confident that eating croutons on her salad had not contributed to weight gain. Her feelings had been real but unreliable. Though we may feel scared to fly or scared of certain foods, we have to remind ourselves of truth. It will help us to face our fears.

What is the first step to recovering from disordered eating and becoming an intuitive eater? You face your fear. You get on the plane. When you face your fear and fly, you may be surprised to find that you'll soar.

You will never reach your destination of making peace with food unless you first take that leap of faith. Face your fear. Get on the plane. Prepare for takeoff. You may feel a little turbulence along the way, but I'm confident you will have a smooth landing.

~ Thirteen ~

PEACE ON EARTH AND PEACE WITH FOOD

Recently, I came across a picture of Santa Claus with this quote: "No more cookies, please. If you don't leave me celery sticks and cucumber water, all you'll get is coal."

This quote describes our culture well when it comes to food. We tend to have an all-or-nothing approach to eating. It's either all the cookies or not even one for Santa.

"Food restriction creates food interest," said Nancy Clark, a registered dietitian.

When Santa restricts himself from eating cookies, he suddenly becomes more interested in cookies than before. Thoughts of cookies consume his mind, which often leads to overeating.

What would happen if Santa had just one cookie and then moved on to the next house? Would he be jollier? Would his red suit fit better? Would his reindeer have less weight to pull in the sleigh?

This holiday season, let there be peace on earth and peace with food.

The holidays are a time to reflect on those things for which we are thankful. They are a time to spend with loved ones and a time to remember the birth of our Savior. For some individuals, the holidays are a time of overeating at holiday gatherings, unwanted weight gain, and unrealistic exercise goals as New Year's resolutions.

Sometimes individuals attend holiday events with rigid food

rules in mind. The challenge occurs when they step outside the boundaries of those guidelines and feel they've broken a rule. This behavior can lead to a "What the heck!" mentality and can trigger overeating.

For example, if you set the rule that you won't have dessert at tonight's holiday gathering, what happens when Nana serves her famous pumpkin pie? If you take only one bite of pie, you'll think you've blown the diet. You may then think, "I've already broken a rule by eating a bite of dessert, so I might as well eat the entire pie."

This overeating often leads to feelings of guilt, more food rules, further restrictions, and eventually back to overeating. The cycle can become vicious and can often lead to weight gain.

We have to make peace with food before we can listen to and nourish our bodies. Making peace with food can help to improve our physical and mental health. It promotes mindful eating and rejects the dieting mentality.

The first step to making peace with food is to consider nothing off limits. Unless you have an allergy, food preference, or medical diagnosis requiring specific food restrictions, all foods can fit into your diet. Remember that food restriction creates food interest, which can lead to overeating.

Allowing all foods to fit into your diet makes the previously off-limit foods less appealing because you know you can take them or leave them. Think of the red truck analogy from the previous chapter. Sound familiar?

A patient once told me she didn't understand how her roommate could eat one cookie and be done. This particular patient would try to eat just one but would end up consuming the whole container of cookies. Each time she ate cookies, she believed it was the last time she would ever eat cookies. Therefore, she overate every single time.

You may have heard the saying, "Eat and be merry, for tomorrow we diet." Many dietitians refer to this as the Last Supper mentality. Over time, this attitude leads to weight gain.

While making peace with food, we need to be aware of the food police. The food-police mentality exists when we make rigid dieting rules and decide what we should or should not eat. This attitude can ignite rebellious eating and overconsumption of food. It makes us feel good or bad, depending on what we have eaten. It makes eating a moral dilemma.

Food is neither good nor bad, and a person is neither good nor bad for eating a particular food. Making eating a moral situation can be dangerous.

Remember to listen to your body by eating when you are hungry and stopping when you are full. This is a lot easier said than done. Remember the difference between physical hunger and emotional hunger. The same dietitian who taught me the red-truck analogy also taught me about tank A and tank B

Tank A is your stomach. That's where food goes. Tank B is your heart. That's where your emotions go. When you are physically hungry, you fill up tank A with food and go about your day feeling better. However, when you have an emotional hunger and shove food into tank B, the tank will still be empty.

Don't forget to show yourself compassion. The goal is progress, not perfection. This may look like taking two steps forward and one step back, but it is still a net step forward. This holiday season, let there be peace on earth and peace with food. Learn what it means to nourish your body and enjoy the pleasures of eating at the same time.

Remember that, with this way of eating, Santa can have his cookies and eat them too. And so can you!

~ Fourteen ~

SAFE AND FUN FOR THE WHOLE FAMILY

Everywhere we turn, we see a billboard advertisement, magazine article, or television commercial marketing a new weight-loss product. Whether it's a pill to pop, a wrap to wear, or a juice to cleanse, we've seen it all.

Each message screams, "You're not good enough," "You're not thin enough," or "You're not pretty enough." They offer false promises to make you happy and trick you into believing that, if only you could shed that stubborn belly fat, all would be right in the world. You'd be happier. Life would be easier. People would like you.

The quick solution to your misery is in a bottle. Just a dose of this and a drop of that for ninety-five dollars a month, and you'll be on the road to success. So you give in and buy a bottle. You pay your dues, order your supplements, and follow meal plans that have you eating bland salads and drinking juices that make you feel as if you're prepping for a colonoscopy.

Your food tastes like a freshly mowed lawn, you have explosive diarrhea, and you feel miserable. That must mean the plan is working, right? Surely you couldn't enjoy your food and still lose weight. That's unheard of.

I'd like to think the Christian radio station would give us a nice break from the negative noise. To my surprise, even they have succumbed to the societal pressures of diet culture. I hear advertisements for Sona MedSpa, Slim for Life, and unwanted hair removal.

As I continue to listen, it gets worse. "Children join free with a parent's enrollment." I must have heard this wrong. Now we are getting kids involved? Why? So we can raise a whole new generation of people who hate themselves, hate their bodies, and have an unhealthy relationship with food?

I continue to listen, hoping it will get better.

The Christian station plays songs about Jesus and His love for us. They sing about abounding grace and our hope being in Christ. The message is short-lived because, just as soon as it came, it's gone, and I'm left listening once again to ways I can lose thirty pounds in thirty days and tips for permanent hair loss in unwanted places.

Then I hear it. The claim. The motto. "Safe and fun for the whole family." Seriously? I appreciate the station's dedication to playing songs with encouraging lyrics instead of foul language, but are these commercials safe and fun for the eight-year-old girl in the backseat who's starting to realize she doesn't have a thigh gap like the other girls in her dance class?

Is it safe or fun for the ten-year-old boy who recently overheard his pediatrician telling his dad that he's over the eighty-fifth percentile, and his eating needs to be monitored more closely? Is it safe for the eighteen-year-old on her way home from an eating-disorder treatment facility and is now trying to figure out how to transition back to the real world?

It's neither safe nor fun. It's confusing. It's conflicting. First I hear that Jesus loves me, that I'm made in His image, and that He knows the numbers of hairs on my head. Then I hear that, if I struggle with value or self-worth, all I need is to slim down or bulk up in order to feel better about myself.

The truth is that no diet plan, no pill, no juice, no wrap, and no monthly subscription will make me feel worthy. No number, no size, no measurement will define my identity.

My hope is built on nothing less
Than Jesus' blood and righteousness;
I dare not trust the sweetest frame,
But wholly lean on Jesus' name.
On Christ, the solid Rock, I stand;
All other ground is sinking sand.

Sinking sand. Diet plans. Pill boxes. Juicers. Wraps. Sinking sand. Finding my worth and identity in the numbers on the scale. Sinking sand.

I may feel good temporarily. I may appear happy for a moment. But eventually, I'll sink. Lower and lower. Deeper and deeper.

Proverbs 31:30 tells us that charm is deceptive, and beauty is fleeting.

Psalm 139:13-16 tells us that God knit us together in our mother's womb. It says that we are fearfully and wonderfully made and that God not only saw our unformed bodies, but He also knew all the days of our lives before one of them came to be.

Some of you may be reading these scriptures for the first time. I pray that your heart receives this truth. Others have heard these verses time and time again in church. Don't brush them off, disregarding their weight. These words have the power to transform our lives.

You might wonder why I've dedicated an entire chapter to the discussion of radio commercials. The reason is the danger of sending our kids mixed messages about the character of God and their identity as His children.

We have to send consistent messages to the next generation. This communication can start in the backseat of the car while the children listen to the radio. We must raise our children to be critics of the media and diet culture, to question what the world tells us and to cling to truth. You can't cling to something you don't know, so we have to know it and teach it to them. It may be the most important thing we do here on earth.

I want to raise up a generation who believes scriptures like Proverbs 31:30 and Psalm 139. Imagine how many fashion industries, diet programs, weight-loss surgery centers, and cosmetology institutes would go out of business if we only lived as if we believe these words.

I want to see a generation that knows there's no solid ground to stand on in this world except Christ, and all else is fleeting. Sinking sand.

In her book *Life Without Ed,* Jenni Schaeffer says, "As long as people like you are becoming educated about eating disorders and are reaching out for help, I believe that young children today can grow up in a society that focuses more on health than on weight—a world that does not consider appearance to be the most crucial aspect of identity. Tomorrow's girls (and boys) might not have to wage wars against their bodies, because we are making changes to ourselves today. Right now."

Just today, I heard a woman say that the devil is strategic in his schemes because he wants to take us down. Therefore we must be strategic as well. I beg of you, please do not sit on the sidelines, waiting for someone else to handle this issue. The time is now.

May we be the hands and feet of Jesus, and may we teach the next generation to walk in the freedom Christ has called us to. Let the lies be silenced and the darkness overcome by light. Let our children know they are God's holy workmanship, created in His image.

Now that is safe and fun for the whole family.

~ Fifteen ~

AM I ENOUGH?

This spring, I attended a women's conference at my church where we heard many well-known Christian women speaking the truth in love from the book of Proverbs.

At the conference, Jada Edwards, author of *The Captive Mind: Evicting Old Thinking to Experience New Life*, spoke on the dangers of transposing truth. Changing truth, even just a little, makes it no longer truth, she said. She gave the example of trying to use her debit card to make an online purchase but accidentally switching two of the numbers when attempting to make the transaction. "Amazon isn't going to respond, 'Well that was a good try, and the card number was close enough so we will go ahead and give it to you.'"

That'd be crazy! Switching only two numbers makes the entire card number invalid, and the transaction cannot be completed. Even the slightest alteration makes something not true, but false.

This scenario is no different than changing the truth, hoping it will sound better or meet our desires. Messing with truth this way is dangerous.

Jada spoke on the importance of knowing the truth of God and recognizing what is not truth. Some quotable and re-tweetable ideas are not truth.

Many things sound good but are not truth. For example:

You are the hero of your story
Love is love

Follow your heart
All roads lead to the same destination

In the eating-disorder treatment realm, I often hear, "You are enough." This sounds great. It looks pretty on a coffee mug or a t-shirt or on the cover of a journal.

We say it in passing as means of encouragement and to build one another up. We tattoo it on our wrists and use it as our motto. We long for it to be true, and we want others to believe it for themselves as well.

You are enough. But are we?

You see, if we were enough, we wouldn't need Jesus. The gospel, in its entirety, would be meaningless. Why would a savior need to come and rescue the world if we are enough?

We are, in fact, *not* enough. And that's okay. We were never made to be enough. God meets us where we are, and through His son, Jesus, He provides our enoughness. We are not enough. He is. That is the whole point of the gospel.

At first glance, it seems depressing to realize that you aren't enough. However, with a new perspective, it is freeing. I can stop trying so hard to be enough because Jesus is enough and so I can walk in freedom.

In her book *Nothing to Prove: Why We Can Stop Trying So Hard,* Jennie Allen says, "I am not enough. And I am done trying to be. God already knows we are not enough, but He's not asking us to be. To get to the place where God can be enough, we have to first admit that we aren't."

This is where it gets good. Allen says, "It's not my curse that I believe I am not enough; it's my sin that I keep trying to be." Mic drop!

If we spend our time and energy in trying to be enough, we lose sight of what God has in store for us and His purpose for us.

What if we stopped looking for our enoughness in a number on the scale, a dress size, or a workout plan and instead rest in the fact that we are not enough, but He is? What if instead of telling people they are enough, we pointed them to Jesus, the one who is enough?

You are not enough. This phrase may not sell mugs or t-shirts, but it's the truth. You are not enough, and that's okay. You were never meant to be enough. Believing Christ is enough for us; we can walk in the freedom He offers. Then we can stop running and trying and doing and performing.

As Jennie Allen says, "I am not enough. And I am done trying to be."

~ Sixteen ~

BABIES AND BODIES

I recently read an article titled "What You'll Miss About Being Pregnant." At thirty-eight weeks pregnant, it's hard to believe I'll miss anything, considering I now waddle like a penguin, spend more nighttime hours in the bathroom than in the bed, and wear a belly-support band to do a load of laundry. Not to mention dropping a dirty sock and taking five minutes to get it off the floor and into the washer.

However, I am grateful for a healthy, safe, and smooth pregnancy thus far. I'm thankful for a willing and able body that can carry and nourish a child. Little waves of movement in my belly remind me of the precious life we will soon get to meet.

The article said a mother might miss the baby's kicks when she is no longer pregnant. I can see that being the case, considering there is something special and intimate about feeling this little guy squirm around and get a case of the hiccups almost nightly. I so treasure these precious moments of my husband placing his hand on my belly and feeling his son bouncing around, almost as if we are getting a glimpse of his little personality before he makes his entrance into the world.

These days, some of my baby's movements feel more like a punch to the gut, an uninvited guest, or an alien invasion to my body. Nonetheless, I could see how I might miss these moments.

One line in this article struck a nerve with me: "You'll miss eating whatever you want." This sentence sends an unspoken message that, under usual circumstances, we should not eat whatever we want, and that pregnancy is our free pass for eating foods we enjoy.

I find it sad. Some people believe the cultural lies that say we can savor foods only on particular occasions or during specific seasons of our lives, such as pregnancy.

Our society fears that, if we allow ourselves to eat whatever we want, we'd contribute to the obesity epidemic. People don't usually stop to consider a different cause: because we don't allow ourselves to eat whatever we want, we do contribute to the obesity epidemic by triggering the Last Supper mentality, binge-eating episodes, and other unnatural, disordered behaviors.

The article mentions the idea of not feeling guilty after eating when you're pregnant. This idea hints that, at other times in our lives, eating is a moral situation, and feeling shame for eating a bad food is the cultural norm. Why does this have to be the case?

The principles of intuitive eating result in the satisfaction of finding pleasure in our food. Research shows we tend to eat less when we find satisfaction in our meals. I think there's something to that.

Part of intuitive eating is also learning to listen to and honor our body's internal cues while properly responding and nourishing ourselves. This concept is part of body respect and self-care, not the "If I eat whatever I want, I'll just let myself go" mentality our society often believes.

The article continues to list things you'll miss, like playing the pregnancy card. I admit to recently taking advantage of this. I now wonder why I waited so late into my pregnancy to use this magical tool. I think my pride got the best of me as I tried to do everything on my own. I wanted to prove to myself and to others that I was as capable and active as I had always been.

Then one night, I tried out this card on my husband by

asking him to get me something to drink from the kitchen. I didn't do this because I couldn't do it myself or didn't feel well, but simply because I was testing the waters with this card. And just like that, a drink appeared, and I didn't have to lift a finger. Magical! With only two weeks left until my due date, I now end most sentences to my husband with, "…but I'm pregnant." So yes, I'd say I'll miss this part of pregnancy. I hear there is a mom card you can play too, so I'm looking forward to that.

One line impacted me more than the rest in this article: "One of the things you will miss about pregnancy is body confidence." I had to re-read this to make sure I had seen it correctly. Unfortunately, I had.

I have spent twenty-three years of my life at war with my body. For the majority of my time on earth, I have not practiced body kindness, body respect, or appropriate self-care. I have fought to alter my appearance, change my shape, and control the number on the scale.

With a lot of work, growing, learning, and immersing myself in the professional field of eating disorders, I have come to a peaceful place with my body. Thankfully, I've remained there for the past six years.

Of course, I initially felt fear when I found out I was pregnant. "How will I respond emotionally to my rapid body changes?" "Will this pregnancy hinder my current relationship with my body?"

Though it hasn't always been easy to observe the rapid body changes that take place during pregnancy, this experience has been more positive than I would have imagined. I've gained more than just pregnancy weight; I've also found a true appreciation for what my body can do and for the fact that it is working for me, never against me.

In some regards, my body confidence has continued in pregnancy. However, this doesn't have to end when a woman has her baby. Who says you should miss being confident in your body after pregnancy? Why not continue to be confident in the amazing truth that your body knows how to adjust slowly to a non-pregnant state by shrinking the uterus, adjusting hormone levels, and now producing breast milk. Our bodies are miraculous and wonderfully created for carrying a baby in pregnancy.

Yet, as soon as the baby is born, we forget all our bodies have done for us. We switch gears and immediately say, "I've got to get my pre-pregnancy body back." or "I hate these stretch marks." or "My boobs aren't as perky as they used to be." Maybe the girls hang a little lower than you'd like these days, but my goodness, they nourished a child on their way down. How amazing is that?

It's as if pregnancy is an amazing body experience, and then the clock strikes twelve, the baby is born, and we go back to bashing our bodies and hating ourselves. We quickly forget what our bodies just did for us and how God created us.

I am not naïve enough to think I don't have a lot to learn. After the birth of my son, I'll meet obstacles that will challenge my thoughts and beliefs about my body. If I am not careful to take those thoughts captive and replace them with truth, I could quickly go back to an all-too-familiar place of self-loathing and body bashing.

I intend to take each postpartum day as it comes and to continue caring for myself by nourishing my body and participating in joyful movement. Caring for myself may take on a different form during my new season of life, but I'll continue to make self-care and mental health my priorities.

I was at Target last week, picking up a couple items on the hospital packing list our childbirth instructor gave us. (I wonder how many first-time moms like me take this all too seriously,

and then by the time the next child comes, we wait until labor
to throw a bag together.)

I came across the women's clothing section, filled with
bright springtime colors and adorable ruffled lace blouses. Now
that I have only about four maternity outfits that still fit comfortably, I was tempted to stop and browse and pick up a couple
new items for summertime.

I decided this might not be the best thing to do, considering that I might not wear the same size postpartum. I soaked
in the truth that my body may settle in a little different place or
weight than it did prior to my pregnancy.

I decided waiting would be better for my mental state and
emotional wellbeing. I resolved to see what my body does after
labor and then, one day, head back to the store and shop for that
body, not the body I used to have or hope to have.

So as tempting as it was to stop and browse, I kept sorting
through the less-than-sexy wireless nursing bras and then
headed to the aisle where the Depends are kept. Oh, how life
has changed.

My pregnancy is drawing near an end, and I am close to
meeting my little baby boy. I'm excited, scared, nervous, and experiencing all the feels at this point. I'm grateful for a smooth
and healthy pregnancy and hope for a safe delivery.

I am also optimistic. I hope to step into this new season of
life and motherhood with a healthy mindset. I plan to allow myself to eat whatever I want in a way that honors my body's crav-
ings and nourishes me. I'll have a new respect for my body and
what it has done for me. And I'll enjoy a humble body confidence that outlasts forty weeks of pregnancy and continues to
the next phase of life.

~ Seventeen ~

FAMILY PATTERNS

Our church is currently in the middle of a sermon series called Family Patterns. On Sunday, my preacher said we can either reflect or reject certain patterns from our childhood as we form our own family and start new traditions.

I began thinking about my childhood experiences surrounding food and the body. Which of those experiences do I want to reflect, and which do I want to reject? I grew up in a food-neutral home, where food was neither good nor bad, and no one dieted. My family sat together at the dinner table most nights and shared a home-cooked meal over conversations about our day. I hope to reflect my mom's compassion for others and her encouraging words of affirmation. I always found a handwritten note on the napkin she'd tucked away into my lunch box. Some of those napkins still sit in a box of keepsakes, worn and torn and crinkled.

As I am now raising a family of my own, I intentionally reject speaking self-criticism. I work hard never to talk negatively about myself in front of my family.

My mom was always hard on herself and had trouble seeing all the positive attributes we saw in her. I never remember hearing her say anything positive about her body. She complained about her hair and criticized her legs. She hid spider veins under pantyhose and her stomach under a girdle.

As a child, I remember comparing myself to her. I wondered that if she thought negatively about her own body, what should I think about mine?

My husband and I are also intentional about not com-
menting on the appearance, size, or shape of others.

My dad is a great man. He's funny, easy to talk to, a leader,
and a follower of Christ. I hope to reflect those qualities. He
never said much about his own appearance, but at times he
commented negatively about other women. He believed ladies
in larger bodies were lazy and gross, and he often made remarks
about girls he viewed as fat, either on television or out in public.
He thought that weight was something everyone could fully
control. He also saw weight as an indicator of health.

One night, my dad told my sister and me that the key to a
happy marriage was for a wife to keep her body in shape, as he
believed my mom had kept hers. I associated size with love and
believed there was a direct correlation between my weight and
the acceptance of others.

Don't get me wrong; my mom and dad have been my
biggest fans. But, as you can see, even parents are victims of the
diet culture and society's thin ideal.

In my office, parents have asked me if they should lock their
refrigerator or cabinets to control their child's eating. (The answer is absolutely not.) In my job, I've heard of parents restricting their children's intake due to the fear of having an
overweight child.

From a young age, these kids were taught not to trust their
bodies to tell them when they were hungry or full. Therefore,
they grew up with a mind-body disconnect, a diet mentality, and
a fear of the word fat.

I've met with a young teenager who asked her mom for a
piece of candy. Before answering, her mom made her stand on
the scale. Depending on her weight, she would or would not get
the candy. Worse, the girl sometimes had to watch her sisters eat
while she got nothing.

I worked with another young teenager who went with her mom to Jason's Deli for a meal pass. A meal pass is given when a patient is allowed to leave treatment to practice having a meal with family in a real-life food scenario. She knew her meal plan called for dessert at dinner. She had high levels of anxiety at the thought of eating ice cream after her meal.

Looking for support, she asked her mom to eat a serving of ice cream with her. Sadly, her mom responded, "I can't. My body is different than yours. If I eat ice cream, it will turn to fat." As you can imagine, this only increased the girl's anxiety.

Just today, I received an email from a thirty-eight-year-old patient whose mom brought up her weight in a recent conversation. The mom asked her to consider weight-loss surgery since nothing she had done in the past had "worked." The patient said none of her previous attempts to lose weight had worked in the past because they all had aimed at fixing the result of the issue instead of addressing its cause. She knew surgery would not fix the underlying emotional triggers that drove her eating behaviors.

Parents often come to me exhausted and overwhelmed. Their child's eating disorder has taken over and has called the shots for far too long. This situation leads to an interruption of family meals, increased conflict, and confusion regarding the proper way to support their loved one.

Many times, parents carry guilt and shame as an unnecessary burden, believing they caused their child's eating problems. If you've read my experience and the experiences of others above, you might think the same.

The truth is that we are all broken people living in a broken world. Someone once said, "Genetics load the gun, but environment pulls the trigger."

Many variables, such as genetic predisposition, temperament, and a history of trauma, can increase the risk of developing an eating disorder. But just as a loaded gun can cause protection or harm, so can one's environment.

Many people don't know how to nourish and care for their bodies properly because no one taught them how when they were children. Many parents want to support their kids in the area of food and body but don't know how. Often, parents innocently cause harm when they're simply trying to help.

Cynthia Culver, Licensed Professional Counselor, says parents often have good intent but poor execution.

I tell parents all the time that they have the opportunity to be a positive example and model a healthy relationship with food and body for their kids, even if they don't have it all figured out themselves.

Our actions speak much louder than our words. When we diet, our kids see. When we body check and critique ourselves in the mirror, our children are watching.

Culver says actions speak louder than words and that kids know exactly what their parents think of their own body as well as their child's, whether or not the parents have commented on the matter.

When we associate weight with worth, we teach the next generation to do the same.

Change starts in the home. Let us teach our kids to be critics of diet culture and the media. Let's enlighten them that their character has much more value than their pants' size and that things like integrity, sense of humor, and loyalty are more important than a number on a scale. As my preacher said on Sunday, we can either reflect or reject patterns from our childhood, depending on whether they were positive or negative experiences.

I used to fear becoming a parent because I believed I might

mess up my kid. The truth is that we are all messed up. Sometimes our kids will just have to struggle and learn through the process with our love and support.

Because of my awareness of the dangers of diet culture and the prevalence of disordered eating, I can be a strong force in my home for promoting body confidence and self-trust. And so can you. By reading this book, you're already equipping yourself more than you know.

You want to be your children's role model for having a healthy relationship with food and body. You want to raise kids who are confident in their bodies and who know their worth is not in their appearance.

But you still don't know how to feed them, right? Do I just let them eat whatever they want? Do I buy only healthy foods? Do I lock the refrigerator? (Again, don't lock the refrigerator.)

Though this book is not meant to be a how-to, I highly recommend checking out the book *Child of Mine* by Ellyn Satter, MS, RD, LCSW, BCD. In her book, she discusses the division of responsibility in feeding, which teaches parents that their role is to decide the "what, when, and where" of eating. The child's role is to determine the "whether" and "how much."

The goal of this model is to help empower children to become competent eaters and to instill body trust. This approach teaches parents how to take into consideration their child's food preferences without catering to all their requests and becoming a short-order cook. It has proven to prevent picky eating and the development of eating disorders.

Remember, it starts at home. What do you want your family pattern to be? Maybe you look back on your childhood and quickly decide what you want to reflect or reject. Perhaps you fear you have reflected many negative attributes and worry that you've caused harm. It doesn't have to be this way. It's not too late to make changes and to model a healthy relationship with food for your children.

Kids are like sponges. They absorb everything. When it comes to how they view their own body and what they think of food, they will either learn something from you or our culture. Don't let the culture teach them.

Be the example. Don't merely tell your children that they are fearfully and wonderfully made. Also show them in the way you behave and in the way you treat your own body.

They are always watching. What do you want them to reflect? Remember, it starts at home.

~ Eighteen ~

HUMMINGBIRD

One of the things I love most about being a dietitian is giving people the freedom to eat and to enjoy what they are eating. I often meet with people who have experienced a lifetime of dieting and had negative childhood experiences, which have shaped and molded the way they now view food.

I recently met a woman who told me she has been on and off diets since she was eight years old. She is now sixty-five years old. After one failed weight-loss surgery, she came to my office, viewing a surgical revision as her last hope of ever experiencing weight loss or a happy life.

I explained to her that another surgery would not heal her aches and pains. I dug into her childhood to get a better understanding of her and discover where her lifelong history of dieting may have originated.

It turned out that her parents started making remarks about her weight and eating behaviors early on. When she was a little girl, her siblings were allowed a dip of ice cream in a large, crunchy cone while she was told she could choose only low-fat sherbet.

She stated that, to this day, when she visits her now eighty-eight-year-old mother, she prefers to eat alone instead of sharing a meal with her to avoid more hurtful words at the dinner table.

Most of my patients don't realize how deeply rooted some of their food-related issues are until they begin unpacking and processing childhood experiences. They come into my office merely looking at their food behaviors. But often, these behaviors are just symptoms or byproducts of an underlying emotional trigger.

As we began to unpack her childhood, she said that when she was a little girl, she used to get so excited about dinnertime that she sat in her chair at the kitchen table and hummed a tune before the meal. What a delightful child she must have been. Unfortunately, her parents did not see this as delightful in the least. They scolded her for getting so excited about eating.

They were concerned about her weight and eating behaviors. The last thing they wanted, or so it appears, was for their little girl to enjoy the food set on the table before her.

For years, this woman was told she was fat. For years, she felt unloved and unaccepted by her parents. For years, she tried one diet after another only to see them fail her, and yet somehow, she felt as if she was the one failing.

She could never have resolved these issues by going under the knife in an operating room for weight-loss surgery. Bariatric surgery transforms the stomach, not the heart. If emotional triggers caused her eating behaviors, the emotional triggers would continue to be there, even if her stomach's capacity for food had significantly decreased.

Physical hunger didn't drive her eating; emotional hunger did. Surgery would not change that. This woman had lost hope and was counting on a revision to her previous surgery as her last saving grace. She wanted a gastric sleeve, when, in some ways, what she needed was a "heart transplant."

I looked the woman in the eyes, her face still reflecting the disappointment of her past. "I want to help you hum again."

A glimmer of hope shone on her face, almost as if a shackle had broken. She was encouraged as we talked about the ideas of working to separate food and feelings and making peace with her plate. We talked about the concept of rejecting the diet mentality and learning to cope with emotions without using food.

She loved the idea of legalizing all foods and learning how to listen to her body to appropriately nourish herself, letting her body weight adjust itself accordingly. At last, she would no longer be a slave to the scale.

At the end of the appointment, we discussed our next appointment time and our plan. I recommended a book that would help her on a new path to intuitive eating.

I walked her out to the main lobby of the office and told her to give me a call if she had any questions or concerns prior to our next visit. She was appreciative of my time, and I think I walked away more encouraged by meeting her than perhaps she was from meeting me.

If you have experienced a lifelong history of dieting and you're tired of hating your body and viewing food as the enemy, this chapter is for you. If childhood experiences have negatively impacted your relationship with food, this chapter is for you. If you haven't truly tasted food in years, this chapter is for you.

I want to help you hum again.

~ Nineteen ~

TWIRLING OUT OF CONTROL

"I wouldn't have been able to twirl," she said under her breath, her gaze dropped, shoulders slumped low in disappointment.

Karen was a middle-aged woman being treated for anorexia nervosa. She had an extensive history, including gastric bypass surgery ten years ago. Many of her eating behaviors and weight-related issues stemmed from adverse childhood experiences, much like many other people who struggle with disordered eating.

During treatment, Karen was blindly weighed each morning, which means she would step onto the scale backward. When an individual has an eating disorder, knowledge of their weight can often trigger problems. One morning, while being blindly weighed, Karen accidentally saw her weight.

"All I could think about when I saw my weight was that I would not have been allowed to twirl." Karen explained that she had been a dancer in high school. Each week, members of the dance team stepped on the scale to see whether or not they would be allowed to perform. Their weight, not their talent, determined their position on the team.

Sadly, this would be the first of two similar stories I would hear within a month. Both women were still scarred from the traumatic event of having to weigh in before a performance.

Although Karen was severely malnourished with sunken cheeks and in dire need of weight restoration, all she could think about was the lie she believed all those years: she was not

76

enough because of her weight. The number on the scale was not simply a relationship between her body and gravity—it was her identity.

No one told her good dancers are strong, graceful, dedicated, or artistic. Instead, her coach told her good dancers were small, thin, and didn't take up much space. So Karen strived, day after day, to control her weight while everything else in her world felt out of control.

Mandy was a woman in her thirties who had been sexually abused. She, like Karen, was being treated for anorexia nervosa. This was her first time to seek help for her eating disorder, a disease she had battled for the majority of her life. Mandy thought if she could be as small as possible, she would somehow disappear. Then she would be unseen, untouched, and finally safe.

Michelle was a wife, a professional, and a mother of two. Her parents taught her to be small and unseen. They scorned her for her vibrant, loud personality. She learned that being quiet meant being small, and this was best. So she worked tirelessly to control her dietary intake and to keep her weight down.

Tina was a transgender male to female struggling with gender identity and feeling unable to express herself. To Tina, being thin meant being feminine, so she strived to be as skinny as possible. She was unable to wear makeup, paint her nails, or dress in women's attire, so she resorted to the one thing she felt she could do: lose as much weight as possible. Then, maybe she would finally feel at peace with her identity.

Many different people, many different stories, but there was one common theme: striving for thinness in order to solve deeper-rooted issues. Each thought a certain body size or shape would make life easier, more manageable.

Karen believed that if she were smaller, she would be accepted, valued as a dancer, and that would be enough. Mandy thought that if she chased the thin ideal, she would ultimately be safe and in control. Michelle decided that if she lost weight, she would finally be the person her parents wanted her to be— quiet and behind the scenes. Tina believed that being skinny would help her somehow to find her true self.

When life feels out of control, it's tempting to grasp desperately for something we think will calm the chaos. A striving for thinness can easily become a way to escape from uncomfortable emotions instead of coping with them. It is easier to have a "weight" problem than a self-worth issue, trauma we haven't resolved, or an unsettledness in gender identity.

Achieving a specific body size or shape will never solve these problems. When anxiety is high, we may reach to dietary restrictions, compulsive exercises, or other forms of disordered behaviors in order to bring the anxiety back to baseline, where it feels more manageable. But this works only temporarily. It's like trying to place a Band-Aid on a gaping wound. Eventually, the anxiety returns at a higher level than before. Food, or a lack thereof, will not fix a broken heart. No number, pants' size, or shape will heal our hurts.

Using eating disorder behaviors to cope with life's struggles only keeps us in the dark, isolated, and ashamed. We must choose healing over hiding, stepping into the light to begin mending what was broken. Only then will we stop twirling out of control.

~ Twenty ~

MATTERS OF THE MIND

Watch your thoughts
For they become words.
Watch your words
Because they become actions.
Watch their actions
Because they become habits.
Watch your habits
Because they become your character.
Watch your character
For it becomes your destiny.
—*Frank Outlaw*

"Just stop thinking about it." If I had a dollar for every time my husband said this to me, I'd be one wealthy woman. You can't sit down and relax because there are dishes in the sink? Just stop thinking about it.

You're mad at yourself for accidentally ruining dinner by forgetting to turn on the crockpot? Just stop thinking about it. Ugh! Nothing pushes my buttons more than those five words.

If only it were so easy to stop thinking about it. Do you think I want to keep brooding over dirty dishes and ruining dinner and having to order takeout? It sounds wonderful to stop thinking about it. But how do I do it?

I'm a thinker, a worrier, an over-analyzer, and a pre-processor. I recently heard a therapist say that a person with anxiety is always thinking "What if" and then dwelling on the worst-case scenario.

That's totally me. What if someone lights a cigarette at the gas station while I'm pumping gas and the whole place blows up? What if that person in the neighborhood isn't merely walking their dog, but is following me like the escaped convict in that episode of Criminal Minds? What if this seemingly mild cough means I'm in the beginning stages of lung cancer?

Most of the time, none of these worst-case scenarios play out, and things transition smoother than imagined. I didn't die during childbirth, the guy was just walking his dog and not stalking me, and the cough cleared up. Most of the time, I worry over nothing.

Do not be anxious about anything, but in every situation, by prayer and petition, with thanksgiving, present your requests to God. And the peace of God, which transcends all under-standing, will guard your hearts and your minds in Christ Jesus (Philippians 4:6-7).

Take captive every thought to make it obedient to Christ (2 Corinthians 10:5).

Did you know that through Christ, we have the power to take our thoughts captive? We don't have to be slaves to our old thought patterns and beliefs. We have the ability to experience a thought, pause, choose not to take the thought for truth, and come up with an alternative one.

Feelings are real but not reliable. I work with many individuals who feel fat or out of control with their eating. Just this afternoon, I met with an eighteen-year-old female who said she feels as if she looks different after drinking water. Therefore, she is scared to drink water.

Feelings are real but not reliable. We have to remind ourselves of truth. I often ask patients to list their eating-disorder rules, thoughts, and beliefs. For example, one rule is not to eat bread because bread will cause you to gain weight.

Many of these patients take these thoughts as truth. They believe that if they eat bread, they will gain weight. Therefore, they give in to urges to restrict their dietary intake. When anxiety is high, they limit the amount of bread they eat. Then their anxiety decreases to a manageable level.

But this pattern of thinking keeps them in the cycle of their eating disorder. They don't take their thoughts captive. Instead, their thoughts take them captive.

It doesn't have to be this way. We can train our brains just as we train our bodies. We can build new patterns of thinking and new habitual behaviors just as we build muscle.

After listing eating-disorder rules, thoughts, and beliefs, each patient lists alternative, healthy self-thoughts. We call this cognitive behavioral therapy. According to the Mayo Clinic, CBT helps you become aware of inaccurate or negative thinking so you can view challenging situations more clearly and respond to them more effectively.

During my sessions with my patient who was scared to drink water, we discussed her rules, thoughts, and beliefs about fluid intake. Her eating-disorder rules told her not to drink water, especially with meals, because she believed she would look different and gain weight if she did.

These feelings were real for her but not reliable. I asked her whether she could look across the room at me and tell whether or not I had just drunk a bottle of water.

She laughed sheepishly and admitted she could not. I told her that, just as a water hose changes shape and becomes firmer when filled with water, so does our gastrointestinal tract. She agreed that this is a normal process of digestion versus an indicator of weight gain. Then we came up with alternative thoughts.

This exercise can help individuals to distinguish between their eating-disorder thoughts and their healthy self-thoughts. Eating-disorder thoughts keep them sick, especially when they act upon those thoughts. Healthy self-thoughts lead to behaviors that align with their values, such as properly nourishing themselves in order to experience an improved quality of life.

We often become victims to our negative thought patterns, believing that if we think something, it must be true. And as the quote at the beginning of the chapter mentions, our thoughts often dictate our behaviors. But Ephesians 4:22-24 tells us we are to take off our old selves and put on our new selves while being made new through changing our attitudes.

I once heard a sermon about renewing our minds and taking our thoughts captive. The preacher told a story about finding mice in his attic. One night, as the preacher and his wife lay down in bed, he heard a rattling noise coming from the ceiling. He discovered mice were living in his attic, so he quickly set traps all around the area.

Night after night, he lay in bed, continuing to hear the rattling of the mice. Then one night as he drifted off to sleep, snap! The trap had caught a mouse. Snap! Snap! Snap! Another and another and another were soon caught in the traps.

The preacher went on to say that in the same way a mouse is caught in a trap, we can learn to take our rattling thoughts captive as we renew our minds. Would you want stinking mice running around your attic? I doubt it. Then why do we let stinking thoughts run rampant in our minds?

As one of my patients says, "That's some stinking thinking!" She's right.

So remember that we can take our thoughts captive. We don't have to fall victim to negative thinking patterns. We can replace lies with truth. To do this, we must recognize lies and know what is real. We can start by getting into the Word to see what is true. We can pray and ask God to give us a spirit of discernment so we can identify lies.

In 2003, the Christian band Casting Crowns released a song called "Voice of Truth." The lyrics declare that I will choose to believe the truth.

The enemy screams out to you. Sometimes it's all you can do to drown out the noise. He's vicious, and his goal is to steal, kill, and destroy.

But oh, the goodness of God! The battle belongs to the Lord, and He has already won. If we take a moment to pause from the busyness and messiness of life, we can hear a gentle, loving whisper that is the voice of truth.

So take your thoughts captive. Challenge your negative patterns of thinking as you do the hard work of renewing your mind. Listen to the voice of truth.

And I pray that the peace of God, which transcends all understanding, will guard your hearts and your minds in Christ Jesus (Philippians 4:7).

~ Twenty-one ~

NON-SCALE VICTORIES

Recently I came across a card at the grocery store that read, "Congratulations on your weight loss!" I nearly stumbled over my grocery cart as I did a double take to make sure I had read it correctly. As familiar as I am with the card aisle at my local grocery store, I had never before seen a card about weight loss.

The card was in a section labeled "Weight Loss," right next to the "Birthday" and "Thank You" sections. It wasn't even categorized under "Congratulations."

Passionate about my career as a non-diet dietitian, I had to do something. But being the passive-aggressive person I am, I couldn't decide whether to buy all the cards to get them out of circulation or steal them so as not to contribute financially to the greeting-card company.

Feeling a little rebellious but not wanting to go to jail for shoplifting a purse full of weight-loss cards, I opted to turn over the first card so no one could see it. I know; it's something a middle-aged mom would do to a card with profanity or nudity on the front. At the time, that was all I had in me. And it felt good. #noregrets

When I got home later that day, I was still bothered that our society places such a strong emphasis on weight and by the message our culture sends us every day: our worth is tied to our weight.

Time and time again, I have met with individuals who have worked tirelessly to make healthy lifestyle changes, break the diet cycle, and move their bodies more. And time and time again, I have sat with these same individuals as they report to me that their weight has not changed, has gone up, or has gone down slower than they'd hoped.

When they tell me about their current weight status, it's as if they'd forgotten their progress. Suddenly, it's all about a number again.

One patient, in particular, had been meeting with me for six months and had worked hard to make peace with food, pinpoint underlying triggers to her emotional eating, and find appropriate coping tools. She also learned to enjoy her eating experience by slowing down and practicing mindfulness.

She came into my office one day after having met with her doctor, her shoulders stooped and her face downcast. Her doctor did not think she was losing weight fast enough. At that moment, she forgot all the progress she'd made over the past half year.

We talked about her lifelong history of restrictive dieting followed by emotional eating and weight cycling. I encouraged her to remember that practicing mindfulness, accepting her body, and making peace with food would be a process. This was not a quick weight-loss fix.

Plus, how had her attempts at weight loss worked for her in the past? Ninety-five percent of dieters regain their weight and have decreased self-esteem, increased anxiety, and increased preoccupation with food.

It was time to try a new approach. This would be a journey, a process, her unique story. She decided to find a different doctor. She would continue to implement the things we had discussed and focus on her non-scale victories.

Non-scale victories are health celebrations unrelated to the number on the scale. In a nutrition class I was teaching one day, I encouraged the participants to think of non-weight-related accomplishments of which they were proud. One lady was proud of herself for finally getting rid of the clothes that no longer fit her comfortably—the "someday" outfits that had hung in her closet for years, reminding her that she was no longer a particular size. They had continued to send her the message that she didn't add up. She decided to get rid of these outfits and to purchase a new wardrobe full of clothes that fit her more appropriately, that complimented her current body and not a future body she hoped to have.

A man said that for him, riding comfortably in an airplane without needing a seat-belt extender was an accomplishment that increased his quality of life. "I call it a non-scale victory," he proudly stated. That was the first time I had heard the term, and I've used it many times since then.

Non-scale victories could be something like achieving the ability to ride a roller coaster comfortably with your child, taking ballroom dancing classes with your husband, playing kickball as a new family hobby, trying new recipes, or practicing self-care. Another non-scale victory could be freely going out to eat with friends instead of eating alone due to fear of ordering from a menu. Non-scale victories can significantly impact your life.

Many variables play a role in our health. Why do we pick our weight as the most important? Wikipedia defines the word "overweight" as having more body fat than is optimally healthy. That is interesting to me, considering that a person in a larger body might eat mindfully, properly nourish their body, and move regularly throughout their day in a way that practices self-care.

However, an individual of normal weight may have irregular and unbalanced eating patterns and lead a sedentary life yet be considered more healthy than the overweight person.

I cannot know anyone's health status simply by looking at their weight any more than I can guess their birthday or how many kids they have.

When life feels out of control, the number on the scale feels like something we can control. However, at the end of the day, we can't control our weight. We can control our behaviors, but the number is going to fall where it will and where our bodies want to be.

A set-point weight is the weight your body naturally wants to be. Our bodies crave homeostasis and work hard to keep us in a place of balance. A set-point weight is the weight at which your body instinctively settles. You don't have to under-eat or over-exercise to maintain this weight.

Interestingly enough, dieting leads to weight cycling (lose, gain, repeat). Over time, weight cycling increases our set-point weight and places us at an increased risk for developing co-morbidities like diabetes and cardiovascular disease.

In her book, *Health at Every Size*, author Linda Bacon, PhD, encourages readers as well as the medical field to consider other indicators of health besides a number. She believes in viewing health from a holistic approach: mind, body, and spirit. She also discusses how behaviors such as eating patterns, mindful movement, and sleep habits are better markers of health.

When we focus on behaviors and let the numbers fall where they will, weight loss sometimes occurs as a result. It's not guaranteed, and it isn't the goal. The goal is behavioral change. This concept doesn't always sell as well, but it works. I've seen lives changed for the better as a direct result.

Non-scale victories. What are yours? Where have you made progress? What non-number-related goal can you work toward?

Maybe you have started eating breakfast daily, breaking your habit of skipping that meal in the past. Maybe your weight hasn't budged, but you've been engaging in movement by taking a fun Zumba class with friends. Celebrate that! Maybe you were able to make it up the parking garage stairs without feeling like a horse pulling a carriage. That's great!

If shifting your focus from a number to behaviors is challenging for you, I encourage you to consider getting rid of your scale for a season. If that step feels too big, think about putting it in a cabinet or closet, away from view. Then you'll have to pause before weighing yourself instead of weighing as an automatic, compulsive behavior.

Many people find it helpful to give their scales to a friend or throw it away. A handful of my patients have found a great thrill in bashing their scales to pieces with a hammer. It can be extremely therapeutic, especially if you've given the scale more control over your life and your worth than it deserves.

I doubt the card aisle of my local grocery store will carry non-scale victory cards anytime soon. Regardless, here is my victory card of encouragement to you:

> You've got this. You don't have to follow the patterns of this world that say your worth and health are based on a number. You can learn, little by little, to make small lifestyle changes, trusting the number to settle at the right place. Go for it. This is your ultimate non-scale victory.

~ Twenty-two ~

BURNED OUT FROM
FEELING THE BURN

I've never been athletic. I've tried every sport, from tee-ball to basketball and from soccer to tennis. I was never tall enough to make the school basketball team. I started at 4'11" with every other elementary-school girl, but they grew taller over the years, and I stayed the same.

I ended up playing basketball for the community because all you had to do was sign up and pay a fee. I made my first basket in my second year and then retired my jersey.

One summer, I went to soccer camp with a friend. She loved soccer and played every season. The community offered a day camp, so I tagged along to see what it was all about.

After the first day, I begged my mom not to make me go back. I used the rainy weather as an excuse, telling her I might be struck by lightning on the soccer field. She bought it, and I stayed home.

I remember trying tennis camp with my sister one summer. She picked it up naturally while I resembled a frazzled girl chasing a fly with a flyswatter.

We tried a change in pace and signed up for English-style horseback riding lessons with a family friend. Our instructor had us line up, one horse behind the other, and follow an obstacle course. While we waited in line, the horse behind me took an interest in my horse's tail, which left me frantically worried that my horse would spook and throw me off.

When it was my turn for the obstacle course, I did not know the routine because I had been preoccupied with the horses' butt situation. My instructor scolded me. That was the last day I ever rode English-style horseback.

I was on the cheerleading squad during my first year of middle school. The second year, we had to try out in front of the entire student body. I opted to be the mascot instead since those tryouts were held in private. They held no risk for public humiliation, that is, until I made it. I got overly excited at one of the football games and tripped over the boys' water bottles. My furry head rolled down the field.

By eighth grade, trying out for cheerleader in front of the entire student body didn't seem so bad. I traded my old, smelly cougar suit, which reeked of Party City and weathered plastic, for a cheer skirt and hair ribbon.

Let's just say that if Jane Fonda VHS tapes counted toward athletics, I would have been voted MVP and would have won the award for the most colorful leotard.

During my freshman year of college, I signed up for a beginner's running class in order to get my kinesiology credit. I had always admired runners but never had it in me to be one. On the first day of the class, the teacher said, "Some of you have been running for years, and others would run only if something were chasing you. This class is for all of you."

I didn't fit into either category. I had run in the past with family members, friends, and off-season girls' athletics. I always pulled the old "I need to stop and re-tie my shoe" trick, which meant, "I can't breathe, so I'm going to take this time to pause and catch my breath as I fumble around with a perfectly tied shoe."

Through hard work, dedication, and perseverance, I have now completed five half marathons, a sprint triathlon, and the

Warrior Dash, which is a three-mile race with obstacles.

For much of my life, exercise was about numbers: calories burned, weight on the scale, and duration and frequency of workouts. The more I focused on numbers, the more joy was sucked out of the activities. It wasn't about doing something social and fun. It was about changing my body and losing weight. It was about punishing myself for the foods I had eaten.

Exercise felt like something I had to do or should do. It was rigid and based on rules. I felt extreme guilt when I didn't work out on a day when I'd scheduled it.

I could miss many morning quiet times in a row without thinking twice, but if I missed one workout, I felt the weight (literally) of it all day. We shouldn't view a quiet time legalistically or feel guilty for missing it, but this goes to show you the condition of my heart.

During pregnancy, I continued to be active but strived to show myself grace in realizing that my changing body couldn't always keep up with my pre-pregnancy routines. I allowed myself to practice mindful yoga or modify specific workouts or walk instead of run (since toward the end of pregnancy, running equaled incontinence).

Now, when I go for a walk with my son in his stroller, I feel joy as I reflect on my blessings and take in the air and the sights around me. The old me would say walking doesn't count and would feel guilty for not running. The new me knows walking is great for my mental health and emotional wellbeing.

Don't get me wrong. I haven't perfected this way of thinking, but perfection was never the goal. I still use my Runkeeper app to track my distance, but I'm not compulsively walking up and down the driveway to get in my last steps.

A few years ago, I met with a man whose doctor had referred him for weight loss. After reading his answers to my list of assessment questions, I realized he was running an average of three hours a day.

When I voiced concern that this was excessive, he said he didn't see it as an issue, since he was still considered overweight. He planned to lose the weight and then figure out what an appropriate amount of exercise looked like.

As the session went on, he divulged that he was struggling in his marriage. Running was the only thing he could do without his wife getting upset. If he wanted to go to a ballgame with his brother or happy hour with his colleagues, his wife got angry, which led to a fight. In a sense, he was running from his marriage. Sadly, this behavior is socially acceptable in today's culture.

If he had been pounding back shots at the bar after work or sleeping with other women, a good friend would ask, "Hey man, is everything okay?" or "What's going on? Do you need to talk to someone?"

However, when someone uses exercise as a way to escape uncomfortable emotions, society views it as admiral and praiseworthy, and the person is considered disciplined and focused.

But the person is still avoiding the underlying emotional issue, which in this case was a struggling marriage. This man traded one maladaptive coping mechanism for another, never dealing with the real problem.

Instead of a meal plan, I recommended marriage counseling. The man stopped showing up to appointments after a few sessions, and I understand why. He wanted someone to validate his disordered behavior, and I wasn't willing to do it.

Doctors might recommend complete exercise restrictions to some people for a season because they are medically unstable or compulsive in their behaviors. I've met with individuals who could not stop exercising. It had become an addiction.

One teenage patient of mine did crunches on the bathroom floor of restaurants. In the treatment center, this patient was placed in a wheelchair to interrupt the behavior.

Others have had trouble sleeping at night because they felt they had to do a certain number of crunches before bed, but they hadn't done them. Some people can't stop running in place in the shower long enough to bathe.

These are extreme cases, but sometimes disordered exercise isn't obvious. Imagine two girls running in a park. They are running the same distance, the same pace, and the same path. One is thinking about the beautiful day. She hears the birds chirping and knows exercise helps her unwind from her stressful day.

The other runner passed on an opportunity to hang out with friends because she knew she'd feel guilty if she didn't work out. She is driven by numbers: miles, steps, minutes, and calories. She runs to make up for lunch or in preparation for tonight's dinner. She runs to change her appearance.

There is a difference between exercise and movement. Exercise is rigid, rule-based, and self-punishing while movement is a mindful, enjoyable form of self-care. It's moving my body because I appreciate it, not because I want to change it.

I've decided to control my activity instead of letting it control me. If we aren't careful, it too can become a bronze snake. I believe activity is a good thing, but it has its place. I think it is good but not a substitute for dealing with underlying emotions.

I believe my body is a temple of the Holy Spirit and that I can honor God by taking care of what He has given me. I also know that, if I'm not careful, I can dishonor Him with my activity due to the condition of my heart.

I am learning, little by little, that my activity tracker, the minutes of my movement per week, and the types of exercise I engage in are not foundational to who I am. My identity has already been set. It is established in the work of Christ, not in any work I do.

Behaviors follow beliefs. I am a child of God, a daughter of the King. If I believe that, I will behave accordingly, whether on the field, the track, or the court.

But let's be real. You won't find me at any of those places.

~ Twenty-three ~

PERFECTLY IMPERFECT

I'm tired. Overwhelmed. Exhausted. I'm done with pretending I have it all together and finished with the façade of having figured everything out.

Early in my career, I worked as an outpatient dietitian at a local hospital, providing nutrition counseling to patients. I preached portion control and mindful eating, and I taught the American Heart Association's recommendations for weekly physical activity. I used my food models—plastic replicas of broccoli, chicken, and pasta—to make a perfectly portioned plate for patients as they sat in my office, desperate for help to make healthy lifestyle changes.

Most evenings, I went home after a stressful day of work and popped in a workout DVD or went for a jog. Then I started dinner, which usually consisted of a balanced meal like the ones on display in my office.

After a while, I grew tired of striving to get it right all the time. I was plagued with feelings of guilt and shame after weekends of traveling or attending events in which I ate past fullness because the food simply tasted so good.

I could never fully enjoy a pizza and movie night with my husband. I felt like a fake, a fraud, a hypocrite. How could I teach people to portion pizza and a side vegetable onto their plate one day and then eat it directly from the box the following night?

One day, after going to the doctor for an annual checkup, I learned that my cholesterol level had become elevated. The doctor prescribed a low-fat diet with increased exercise. I wanted to scream! I wanted to call the office and let them know that, if they'd taken one glance at my chart, they'd have seen that my diet was well balanced, and I was already very active.

With that phone call, I felt discouraged. How was I supposed to help others if the doctor thought I needed help? This constant self-evaluation and criticism led to a decrease in motivation in my career and made getting up for work each day more and more of a challenge.

I had started finding my worth and identity, or lack thereof, in my work. And I believed that if I wasn't doing it perfectly, I wasn't doing good work.

When I began working at an eating-disorder treatment facility, our treatment team consistently taught self-care, self-compassion, and self-curiosity.

Self-curiosity is the opposite of self-judgment. It is getting curious with yourself and asking questions like, "Why did I eat so much today when I wasn't even hungry? Could it have been because I was tired or stressed?"

Self-judgment says, "You shouldn't have eaten so much. You weren't even hungry. You're just lazy and undisciplined, and you'll never figure out this whole food thing." Self-judgment rarely motivates behavioral change.

At the treatment facility, when patients struggled, we reminded them of the goal: progress and not perfection. When they voiced shame over a particular eating issue, we encouraged them to view it as a learning opportunity versus a pass-or-fail situation.

The more I counseled patients in treatment, the more I began to internalize the message I was sharing with them. I started to realize that the most relatable people are often the ones who allow themselves to be human instead of always pretending to have it together. They are the ones who allow themselves to be perfectly imperfect.

I participate in a monthly conference call in which a group of dietitians receive supervision, discuss challenging cases, and provide support to other professionals. During a particularly challenging month, I learned that the next meeting would include a discussion of times when we have felt inadequate as dietitians. What perfect timing!

During the call, we all spoke about times when we felt inadequate and ill-equipped to handle particular clients or situations. I shared my current struggle. For months, I had pressured myself to believe a lie: I had to know it all now, or I wasn't successful.

The facilitator of the call said, "We want to give people answers to their problems. If we can't, or if we can't fix a situation, we're tempted to believe we are the problem. This leads to burnout. The world needs to hear what you have to say, so getting burned out and quitting is definitely not the answer. To prevent burnout, you have to recognize that the problem is not you. The problem is that we don't know what causes eating disorders."

Through that meeting and a lot of self-reflection, I started to realize that God's purpose for my career may have nothing to do with my knowledge of nutrition. It may have nothing to do with the number of credentials behind my name or the number of years I have treated individuals with eating disorders. God's purpose for my career may have nothing to do with me. In fact, by focusing so much on myself, I may have missed His purpose for me.

Perhaps I've been too focused on making a name for myself instead of knowing Jesus and making Him known to others. Maybe God's plan for my job goes beyond nutrition. It could be that this career path is simply a means of displaying the gospel to a watching world.

I'm learning that God has equipped me with compassion and empathy. He is teaching me to be a better listener. He provides me with opportunities to meet people in some of the most vulnerable and darkest times of their lives and to walk alongside them in their process of choosing healing over hiding.

He's teaching me that being a model for others is more than having all the answers. It's more than cooking Pinterest-perfect meals and much more than the amount of activity I've engaged in over the past week. Being a model for others is allowing myself to be an imperfect human and pointing people toward Christ as I follow Him.

I recently attended a conference where a dietitian spoke about the importance of clinicians embracing their own imperfections. He encouraged clinicians to be role models for being imperfect and discussed how professionals can be more relatable when practicing imperfection. In his presentation he said, "Allow yourself to be vulnerable and human. Allow yourself to fail, knowing you failed while trying your best."

This means I don't have to love my body 365 days of the year. I'm allowed to have days when I struggle with my own body acceptance or times when I eat according to underlying emotions. Sometimes I may have to tell a patient, "I don't know, but I'll find out."

In her book *Present Over Perfect*, Shauna Neiquest shares that her striving for perfection in life caused her to miss out on being present with friends and family. Her drive for perfection in her career led to burnout and sadness until she learned the importance of being present for the people we love.

In *Nothing to Prove*, author Jennie Allen shares a similar experience of constant striving followed by numbing out. She describes a cycle of working toward achievement to prove herself to others, followed by seasons of depression and numbness when she realized she wasn't enough.

According to Jennie, we should stop striving for God and instead begin spending time with Him. She also compares the endless exhaustion of attempting to do things on our own with allowing God to equip us for the work He has in store for us.

In a vision, she saw herself getting to heaven one day and seeing warehouses lining the roads of eternity. These buildings stored the skills and tools God was waiting to provide Jennie with if she would only look to Him. In her vision, God whispered to her, "For all that I ever prepared for you to accomplish, I was also waiting to equip you with every single thing that you needed to do it."

When we try to do enough, be enough, and accomplish enough on our own, Jennie says, we're left with nothing but longing in our souls. Her words convict me of my need for desperate dependence on God to work in and through my life.

When we practice being perfectly imperfect, we realize our need for a merciful Savior, and we grow to know and love Him more. When we practice being perfectly imperfect, we allow God to lead and guide us, and we trust Him to place us where He wants us and to equip us for the work He gives us. When we practice being perfectly imperfect, we can experience true joy in our labor instead of burning out from endless striving for achievement and enoughness.

When I choose to be perfectly imperfect, I can make a gourmet dinner for my family or order takeout. I can go for a run or stay home and rest. I can read a nutrition book that increases my knowledge and strengthens me in my career, or I can read a novel while nestled under a blanket on my couch.

In this challenging yet exciting season of my life, I enjoy my job, personal life, and God more by allowing myself to be perfectly imperfect.

~ Twenty-four ~

BODY BULLY

"They used to call me a hippo," she said one day in my office.

"Who?" I asked.

"The other kids at school." This woman was now twenty-eight years old, but she remembered the bullying words that haunted her from her days on the playground.

Kids say the darnedest things, and sometimes there is nothing cute about it. Sometimes their words leave scars that we carry into adulthood, wounds that shape us into who we are or how we view ourselves.

Even worse, at times adults say the darnedest things too. Co-workers comment on our weight, family members mention our need to diet, and strangers whisper hurtful judgments as we pass by.

What happens, however, when we are both victim and bully, and hurtful words come at us from our own inner critic?

"My belly roll is lopsided. If I'm going to have a roll, it should at least be symmetrical." Of all the comments I've heard in my office before, this was a first. It came from a thirty-eight-year-old mother of two.

"It's from my C-section scar. With my second pregnancy, I had to have an emergency C- section or else my son would have died. There was no time to lose, and the doctors cut an uneven line. Not only did this leave a scar, but my belly roll lines the scar and draws more attention to my midsection. I have a lopsided roll."

"What about your son?" I asked. "How is he?"

"He's fine. He's alive and healthy and two years old."

"This lopsided roll sounds like a miracle mark to me," I said. "It sounds as if that scar is a daily reminder of the healthy boy who is alive and well in your home."

She paused. "I never thought of it that way."

We spend too much time bullying our bodies, saying, for example that my legs are too short, my thighs are too round, or my stomach resembles an empty kangaroo pouch. We would never say these things to other people, yet why do we find it acceptable to talk to ourselves this way?

I can only imagine how much it must break God's heart to hear His children cry out against His creation. I firmly believe that the enemy uses negative body image as a distraction, pulling our eyes off God and others and onto ourselves.

Blessings turn into praise of the Father, but burdens rarely do. If I know, understand, and believe in my worth, I'll naturally praise and honor the Father. But if I hate and complain and curse myself, I could end up in a spiral of shame that will keep me in the cycle of disordered eating. The devil knows this and uses it against us.

My sister recently attended my parents' church and said she was at her wit's end that particular Sunday morning. She was juggling an energetic three-year-old with a newborn baby. In addition, she was struggling with putting a house back on the market due to a contract falling through along with an upcoming move from Arkansas to Texas.

She had recently questioned her abilities as a parent and battled with thoughts that maybe she wasn't cut out to be a mom. Some people consider motherhood their life's calling. My sister was starting to feel as if a nap was her life's calling.

The sermon that day taught her that God equips us when

He calls us. He had called her into motherhood and had equipped her with the tools needed for the role. How dare she question whether she was cut out for a role for which God had equipped her? This message not only convicted my sister, but it freed her as well.

It's the same with our bodies. We battle our freckles, our receding hairline, our height, and the size of our nose. Yet God is saying, "I've set you apart. Your body is a temple." And we question it time and time again.

In his book *Victory Over the Darkness*, Neil T. Anderson says of believers, "The body of the spiritual person has also been transformed. It is now the dwelling place for the Holy Spirit and is being offered as a living sacrifice of worship and service to God."

What does it mean for our bodies to be a temple of the Holy Spirit? In the Old Testament, the temple was the dwelling place of God. God's people visited the temple to offer sacrifices and worship to the Lord. But through the work of Jesus on the cross, God now dwells in believers through the Holy Spirit. Our bodies are His temple, and we are told to honor God with them.

Behavior follows beliefs. Anderson says, "The more you reaffirm who you are in Christ, the more your behavior will begin to reflect your true identity."

If I believe my weight makes me unworthy, my size makes me unlovable, or my lopsided roll makes me disgusting, I will behave in a way that reflects that belief. According to Anderson, "Countless numbers of Christians struggle with their day-to-day behavior because they labor under a false perception of who they are."

This behavior could be dietary restriction, abusing laxatives, over-exercising, self-induced purging, and more.

But if I truly believe I am fearfully and wonderfully made

and that my body is a dwelling place of the God of all creation and that He knows the number of hairs on my head and that not one person has my same fingerprint, I cannot help but behave accordingly.

This belief doesn't mean I will never have bad-body-image days or struggle with unwanted thoughts about myself. But it does mean I have the power to question those thoughts and emotions and to remind myself of truth.

As I write this, I have just weaned my son from breastfeeding. Thank goodness this season has ended. I know some women love breastfeeding and others long to do so, but just reread *What They Don't Teach You in Nutrition 101*, and you'll understand.

I was prepared for body changes during pregnancy, and even after birth, but I wasn't prepared for my body to change after breastfeeding. My metabolism has slowed, and my body has settled in a less-comfortable place. Old, unwanted thoughts have popped into my mind like an unwelcome guest. I cover up more, second-guessing myself and pulling at my waistline to adjust my jeans.

I recently saw a picture of a postpartum woman holding two plates over her chest. The comment read, "They may be saggy, but my breasts have fed over a million meals to four children."

We're quick to forget the miracles our bodies indeed are. The fact that my body pushed out a human being should point me to the Creator in an act of worship toward the Father. Yet, instead, it points me to stretch marks, cellulite, and a leaky bladder.

Dear daughter, you are a child of the living God. He knit you together in your mother's womb and knew all the days of your life before one of them came to be. He has made your body a temple of the Holy Spirit and has called you Imago Dei, which means image of God. Let this belief sink in. May it forever determine your behavior.

~ Twenty-five ~

BMI: But My Identity

Last night I attended a networking meeting for eating-disorder professionals. An eating-disorder treatment facility hosted the event at a local theater. We watched a new documentary called "The Student Body." The film was created by a high-school student in Ohio who was challenging a recently-passed bill. The bill allowed schools to weigh students, test their body mass index (BMI), and send home a report card that assessed the student's health status.

BMI is a measurement of body fat based on height and weight. The BMI chart puts you into a weight category: underweight, overweight, obese, or morbidly obese.

The limitations of this measuring instrument include the fact that it takes into consideration only two variables: height and weight. It does not include age, activity level, genetics, eating patterns, muscle mass, or any other relevant factor for determining one's health status.

For example, Arnold Schwarzenegger has a BMI of 33, which places him in the obesity category. Let that sink in for a minute.

Therefore, in my opinion, BMI is just a number. It gives information, but it is far from telling the whole story.

The goal of this bill was to help in the fight against child obesity. At first glance, this looks like an admirable cause. However, through this bill, students in Ohio were sent home with "fat letters" showing where they fell on the BMI chart.

Again, this is all in the name of health. However, shaming

kids over their body size is far from encouraging healthy behaviors. On the contrary, it usually triggers an increased preoccupation with food, which we know can increase the risk of developing an eating disorder.

Furthermore, our nation's approach to solving the child obesity epidemic may instead contribute to it. Traditional healthcare professionals are concerned with the intuitive eating movement because they fear that giving people unconditional permission to eat (which is one of the IE principles) will cause obesity. But we tell people what not to eat, and we have an obesity problem. So maybe food restriction is not the solution.

In this documentary, multiple students were interviewed after receiving their letters. Many were confused, discouraged, and ashamed. Some questioned their own bodies. Parents spoke of their frustration with the school system and their complete sense of helplessness when they saw their child's despair upon opening the letters.

One boy said he didn't understand why he was considered obese when he ate his fruits and vegetables every night. A young girl's family gave a tour of their home garden and discussed their hopes for incorporating gardening into the schools as a way of growing fresh produce for kids' lunches. They were astounded to find that, even though they strive for health and wellbeing at home, their daughter was considered unhealthy according to the school standards.

Fed up with this injustice, the student who created the film spoke with members of legislation about the chaos this bill has caused in her school and in the hearts of her peers. She explained her concern that these letters may do more harm than good in the fight against child obesity. She discusses how BMI testing is not the most accurate indicator of health.

You may think this young student is brave and courageous

for standing up and speaking with legislators, but it gets better. At the end of each interview, she asked each legislator to stand on the scale she brought with her. She then recorded their weight and calculated their BMI.

Most of the legislators refused to weigh in. When held to their own standards, they were unwilling to be weighed.

This brave young girl continued to fight the good fight. Though she faced many obstacles along the way, she persevered. The bill was changed three years later, which was great news for future students.

I've always known BMI is not the best indicator of health. However, we continue to use it both in the healthcare field and the insurance world. I wait in anticipation for the day when this number is no longer used, because I have seen the face of devastation when a patient learns their BMI places them in the category of obese, even after making many positive behavioral changes.

Hearing that you are obese is not motivating. It's shaming and usually leads to self-punishing behaviors that are far from acts of self-care. Therefore, no one learns how to care for himself or herself properly, because they are merely told they are fat and fat is bad.

You don't have to tell someone they are overweight for they are usually well aware of the fact. Stating it does not help the problem, nor does it motivate the individual. Furthermore, you simply cannot determine someone's health status just by looking at his or her weight. I have worked with many overweight individuals who were malnourished, as well as many underweight patients who struggled with binge eating. And placing this much emphasis on weight causes us to look to a number to define our worth.

Like many of the kids in the documentary, a lot of adults

place their identity in the number on the scale, the size of their pants, or the BMI chart at their doctor's office. They let these numbers, rather than their internal cues, dictate their eating behaviors, which further disconnects them from their body. They allow a number to determine whether or not they have a good day and whether or not they are worthy of love.

After the showing of the documentary, we had a question-and-answer session. One dietitian said she was fed up with BMI scores being used as a measurement of health. She called it a "Bulls*** Measuring Instrument."

On my way home that night, I started thinking of BMI as "But My Identity" as a way of stating what my BMI is not versus what it is.

But My Identity is not in the numbers on the scale, whether low after a morning jog or high after a much-needed lunch out with friends.

But My Identity is not in the food I ate for dinner, whether it was a home-cooked, three-course meal at the dinner table or a Little Caesar's Hot-N-Ready in front of the TV.

But My Identity is not in how my wedding gown fits my body after five years of marriage, whether I resemble a Disney princess or a broken can of Pillsbury biscuits.

But My Identity is not in how many minutes I spent being active in a week, whether it was 150 minutes based on the American Heart Association guidelines or if it was 0 minutes because my schedule was packed, and I chose to rest.

But My Identity is not in anything (numbers, scales, weights, measurements, charts, graphs) apart from God.

My identity is in being a child of God, a daughter of the King.

My identity is in being made in His image and being washed in His blood.

My identity is in who Jesus Christ says I am, which doesn't depend on what I can do, but rather on everything He has already done.

This measures extensively more than a number ever will.

~ Twenty-six ~

NEW YEAR, NEW YOU?

As I sit on a plane in the early evening, heading from DFW to NYC for a long weekend with my husband, I'm filled with anxiety and excitement. Anxiety because I hate flying. The last time I flew, I was separated from my husband on the plane. I sat by a middle-aged mom, clinging to her arm as she comforted me while her teenage daughter sat gazing out the window, care-free.

At the same time, I'm excited because I'm visiting the Big Apple for the first time. I can't wait to explore everything NYC has to offer: Central Park, Ground Zero, the Statue of Liberty, and Broadway shows. I look forward to spending my weekend in this great historic place, although "the city that never sleeps" sounds like an insomniac nightmare to me.

When I think about NYC, New Year's Eve in Times Square comes to mind. I love seeing the big ball drop as locals and tourists ring in the New Year. I watch in anticipation of the clock striking twelve with fireworks lighting up the sky, followed by the kisses and cheers of the crowd.

When the ball has dropped, and everyone has gone home, all that remains are empty bottles, trampled confetti, and New Year's resolutions. According to a YouGov poll, the most common aspirations for the coming year in the US are to eat healthier, get more exercise, and save more money.

Along with New Year's resolutions, we hear the familiar chant of "New Year, New Me." This phrase is often played out in the form of restrictive dieting, compulsive, rule-based exercise, and other drastic measures, all in an attempt to change one's size and shape.

Most people do this in the name of health. However, after a while, most people will experience weight cycling (lose, gain, repeat), which increases the risk of developing certain illnesses, such as diabetes and cardiovascular disease, not to mention the toll that restrictive dieting and militant exercise takes on one's mind. Engaging in these behaviors can lead to increased anxiety, depression, and social isolation. It sounds far from healthy to me!

We live in a culture that admires this form of self-punishment and neglects self-care. We praise the woman who can turn down her favorite Danish at the coffee shop and covet the man who finds time in his schedule to hit the gym before, during, and after work. We say things like, "You have such willpower and discipline," and "Nothing tastes as good as skinny feels." We strive to lose ten pounds in ten days or eat "whole" for thirty.

When we can't live up to the unrealistic standards we have set for ourselves, we hide in shame, believing the lie that the problem is us and not the diet. If only we had a little more self-control.

So we vow to tighten the reins even further on our dieting, removing food groups here and there and skipping some meals entirely or drinking them instead. We hit it harder in our workouts and push through fatigue and injuries. The cycle continues, and we discover we are still stuck with our old selves with new aches and pains and fewer carbs in our pantry.

There is a big difference between engaging in behaviors to care for oneself better and engaging in those to change one's appearance. Deciding to add an extra serving of vegetables to my dinner each night to increase my intake of vitamins, minerals, and fiber is different from saying, "I need to lose ten pounds by next month for a big event, and I'm willing to take drastic measures if necessary to reach my goal."

We often set out to change our appearance in the name of "health," all the while engaging in far-from-healthy behaviors.

How do we navigate the ever-rough waters of diet culture?

Let's resolve to give up dieting. Let's resolve to fast from visiting triggering social-media sites and embracing trendy nutrition fads with false claims that are here today and gone tomorrow. Let's resolve to learn the art of body kindness and to do the hard work of healing our relationship with food. Let's resolve to practice mindfulness, size acceptance, joyful movement, and self-care.

This year, let us lay down the mantra of "New Year, New Me." Instead, let's focus on "New Year, Same Me, but Better Cared For." It doesn't have a nice ring to it, but you get the picture. As the current year comes to an end and the new year is upon us, what will your New Year's resolutions be?

Below are some ideas for non-diet and non-scale focused resolutions:

- Find social, enjoyable physical activities to engage in
- Add an extra serving of fruits and/or vegetables to a meal each day
- Aim for eight hours of sleep each night
- Practice one self-care routine daily (reading a book, taking a bath, participating in yoga, journaling)
- Keep a list of words of affirmation for yourself, but only those that are not related to your appearance
- Unfollow triggering social-media sites
- Hide or get rid of your scale if it triggers you
- Practice listening to internal hunger/fullness cues and work to separate food and feelings

• Join a body-image support group
• Read a body-positive book such as *Intuitive Eating,*
    Body Kindness or *Health at Every Size*

This New Year's Day, let's resolve to shift our focus from changing our appearance to changing our mindset. Let's also decide to shift from self-punishing behaviors to self-care practices.

Happy New Year to the new you!

~ Twenty-seven ~

REFLECTIONS

Christ can take your calamities and with the power of the cross, help them make your calling come to be (Chrystal Evans Hurst).

It is February and 74 degrees in Texas. As I sit on my back porch on this winter afternoon, I'm reminded that my life is currently as unpredictable as the Texas weather.

I reflect on where I have been over the past years and where I hope to go, and I am overwhelmed by God's provision and timing. Truly His plans are better than our own.

Seventeen years ago, as a thirteen-year-old girl, I would never have thought my struggle with anorexia would turn into a deep-rooted passion for helping others to heal in their recovery from disordered eating. I never would have thought I would end up following in Carol Park's footsteps and become a dietitian myself.

Seven years ago, I anxiously logged into my computer to find I had not matched with any dietetic internship programs. That day, I never imagined that within a few short months, a new internship program would open in Dallas and would accept me into their charter class.

When I didn't get the job of outpatient dietitian at Baylor Scott and White Health, I may not have believed you if you'd told me I would apply again that same year and then work there for two years while building the outpatient program.

I definitely wouldn't have believed you if you'd told me that, after not getting a second interview at the Eating Recovery Center, the nutrition manager unexpectedly would offer me my dream job the following year.

And on top of all of that, my twenty-year-old self would pinch my thirty-year-old self in disbelief when learning I would build my own private practice specializing in eating disorders, write a book, and develop a speaking ministry, equipping young girls and women to be who God has called them to be.

Below is an excerpt from my journal in October of 2016:

My goals:
• Work fulltime with sufferers of eating disorders
• Write a book
• Participate in a women's ministry for healthy body image
• Impact the lives of young girls

It has been great to watch the plans for my life unfold and to see how God has helped make my mess into my ministry. He has also humbled me along the way by allowing me to stumble every now and then in my own area of eating challenges, body struggles, and anxiety. But it's helped me to relate to the individuals I treat. It also reminds me that I am only human.

This journey hasn't always been easy. I remember being discouraged, tears flooding my eyes, when I asked God why I didn't get into an internship program. I had always thought this was what I was supposed to do. I didn't understand at the time why it felt as if He was keeping me from a desire He had laid on my heart.

It's almost as if He was saying, "Be patient, daughter. You don't know the plans I have for you, but I do. And they're good plans!"

I also felt discouraged when I didn't get the outpatient position at first. I felt stuck in my job at the time, with tons of pent-up passion and a vision, but no idea how to get there.

I cried and stressed and complained about resolving scheduling issues and verifying insurance coverage for patients when it wasn't my job. I didn't know these skills would prepare me to have a business of my own.

I remember driving past the Eating Recovery Center on my daily commute to work and saying, "This is where I want to be." And then one day I didn't pass it. Instead, I drove right to it, parked my happy self in the parking garage, and badged in for my first day. But it wasn't all easy, and the path wasn't always smooth.

In her book, *Kingdom Woman*, Chrystal Evans Hurst quotes an unknown author listing many people with flaws. She said:

Noah was a drunk. Abraham was too old. Isaac was a day-dreamer. Jacob was a liar. Leah was ugly. Joseph was abused. Moses had a stuttering problem. Samson had long hair and was a womanizer. Rahab was a prostitute. Jeremiah and Timothy were too young. David had an affair and was a murderer. Isaiah preached naked. Jonah ran from God. Peter denied Christ. The disciples fell asleep while praying. Zacchaeus was too small. Paul was too religious. Lazarus was dead.

These were all ordinary people God used to do extraordinary things. I think sometimes we assume Bible characters were perfect heroes none of us could relate to. We are so familiar with their story for so long that we miss the point.

When we think of David, we think of him slaying a giant, tending sheep, playing a harp, and being a man after God's own heart. But we forget he had an affair with a woman and then murdered her husband. We know Paul suffered for Christ and wrote letters of encouragement to others while in prison, but we forget he killed Christians for a living before his conversion. If God can use these people for His kingdom, He can certainly use us too.

God took a girl who yearned for a thigh gap and despised her hairline and used her to teach others that worth and identity are not found in appearance. He took a girl with a distorted view of food and a distorted view of herself and taught her what it meant to be made in His image so she might teach others.

If I'm not careful, I can start to build myself up, making more of me and less of Him. I may think, "Look at all I've accomplished," or "What a great job I've done." But when I reflect on the past, I can see clearly through the hard times and the disappointments. God perfectly orchestrated everything in His time and for His glory, not my own.

I don't know where you are in your journey. Maybe everything has turned out as you had hoped it would. Maybe nothing has turned out the way you expected. Maybe you are in a period of waiting or a season of disappointment. But your trust in the Lord is greater than this momentary disappointment.

Today's testing may be tomorrow's testimony. This year's mess may be next year's ministry. Your current calamity may be your eventual calling.

~ Twenty-eight ~

CLOSING THOUGHTS

We've come to the end of our journey together, but in some ways, I hope it is just the beginning for you. Again, this is not another anti-diet or how-to book. You can find a plethora of great resources on the topic of intuitive eating (and the book Intuitive Eating is one of them).

If nothing else, I hope you close the last pages of this book with a changed perspective on food and a new outlook on your body. I hope that within each page, you have read proof that your worth and identity are found in Christ alone, and that this belief transforms every area of your life.

I hope you continue to wrestle until you rest in who God has called you to be. I pray the chains of disordered eating would be broken, and I pray against the lies of the enemy. I pray that you walk in confidence with boldness, knowing your worth is secure in your Creator, and that you courageously live a life set apart for the kingdom of God.

I hope you know you're made in the image of God. I hope this knowledge changes your life when it sinks in that the Creator of all things made you unlike anyone else. He has plans for you and has numbered the days of your life. I hope you know it and believe it and live it out. And I hope it changes the world. Not for our glory but for His.

Go on, dear reader. I am cheering you along the way. May you find worth only in Him for finding it in anything else is nothing but unworthy weight.

About the Author

Kristin is a Certified Eating Disorder Registered Dietitian who owns a private practice in Dallas, Texas, called Wonderfully Made Nutrition Counseling, LLC. Kristin works with individuals struggling with disordered and emotional eating as well as a history of chronic dieting using a non-diet approach.

Kristin holds a degree in nutritional sciences through Texas A&M University. She graduated from Medical City Dallas Hospital's Dietetic Internship Program and later specialized in eating disorders through the International Association of Eating Disorder Professionals. She has experience working in multiple eating disorder treatment centers and treating patients at all levels of care.

Kristin currently serves on the board of the DFW International Association of Eating Disorder Professionals as the Membership Co-Chair. She is a member of the International Federation of Eating Disorder Dietitians, founded the In His Image Body Image Conference for Young Teens and Women, has led women through body image curriculum as part of the Recovery for Life Ministries, and has had the privilege of speaking on the topic of body image and disordered eating at multiple events.

Kristin lives in a small town south of Dallas, called Corsicana. She and her husband have a son with a daughter on the way. They live with their two labs and pet pig, Poppins, on four acres in the country and enjoy being outdoors every chance they can get!

For more information visit:
www.WonderfullyMadeNutritionCounseling.com or email Kristin at Kristin@WondergullyMadeNutritionCounseling.com